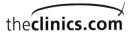

HEART FAILURE CLINICS

Valvular Disease

GUEST EDITOR
Blase Anthony Carabello, MD

CONSULTING EDITORS
Jagat Narula, MD, PhD
James B. Young, MD

October 2006 • Volume 2 • Number 4

SAUNDERS

An Imprint of Elsevier, Inc.
PHILADELPHIA   LONDON   TORONTO   MONTREAL   SYDNEY   TOKYO

W.B. SAUNDERS COMPANY
A Division of Elsevier Inc.

1600 John F. Kennedy Boulevard. • Suite 1800 • Philadelphia, Pennsylvania 19103-2899

http://www.theclinics.com

HEART FAILURE CLINICS
October 2006
Editor: Karen Sorensen

Volume 2, Number 4
ISSN 1551-7136
ISBN 1-4160-3865-5

Reprints: For copies of 100 or more, or articles in this publication, please contact the Commercial Reprints Department, Elsevier Inc., 360 Park Avenue South, New York, New York 10010-1710. Tel.: (+1) 212-633-3813; Fax: (+1) 212-462-1935; e-mail: reprints@elsevier.com.

The ideas and opinions expressed in *Heart Failure Clinics* do not necessarily reflect those of the Publisher. The Publisher does not assume any responsibility for any injury and/or damage to persons or property arising out of or related to any use of the material contained in this periodical. The reader is advised to check the appropriate medical literature and the product information currently provided by the manufacturer of each drug to be administered to verify the dosage, the method and duration of administration, or contraindications. It is the responsibility of the treating physician or other health care professional, relying on independent experience and knowledge of the patient, to determine drug dosages and the best treatment for the patient. Mention of any product in this issue should not be construed as endorsement by the contributors, editors, or the Publisher of the product or manufacturers' claims.

Heart Failure Clinics (ISSN 1551-7136) is published quarterly by Elsevier Inc., 360 Park Avenue South, New York, NY 10010-1710. Months of publication are January, April, July, and October. Business and editorial offices: 1600 John F. Kennedy Boulevard, Suite 1800, Philadelphia, PA 19103-2899. Customer service office: 6277 Sea Harbor Drive, Orlando, FL 32887-4800. Periodicals postage paid at New York, NY and additional mailing offices. Subscription prices are USD 157 per year for US individuals, USD 260 per year for US institutions, USD 54 per year for US students and residents, USD 189 per year for Canadian individuals, USD 292 per year for Canadian institutions, USD 189 per year for international individuals, USD 292 per year for international institutions and USD 65 per year for foreign students and residents. To receive student and resident rate, orders must be accompanied by name of affiliated institution, date of term, and the *signature* of program/residency coordinator on institution letterhead. Orders will be billed at individual rate until proof of status is received. Foreign air speed delivery is included in all *Clinics* subscription prices. All prices are subject to change without notice. POSTMASTER: Send address changes to *Heart Failure Clinics*, Elsevier Periodicals Customer Service, 6277 Sea Harbor Drive, Orlando, FL 32887-4800. **Customer Service: 1-800-654-2452 (US). From outside of the US, call (+1) 407-345-4000.**

Heart Failure Clinics is covered in *Index Medicus.*

Printed in the United States of America.

Cover artwork courtesy of Umberto M. Jezek.

CONSULTING EDITORS

JAGAT NARULA, MD, PhD, Professor, Medicine; Chief, Division of Cardiology; and Associate Dean, University of California Irvine School of Medicine, Irvine, California

JAMES B. YOUNG, MD, Chairman and Professor, Department of Medicine, Lerner College of Medicine; and George and Linda Kaufman Chair, Cleveland Clinic Foundation, Case Western Reserve University, Cleveland, Ohio

GUEST EDITOR

BLASE A. CARABELLO, MD, The W.A. "Tex," Jr, and Deborah Moncrief Professor of Medicine and Vice-Chairman, Department of Medicine, Baylor College of Medicine; Medical Care Line Executive, Veterans Affairs Medical Center, Houston, Texas

CONTRIBUTORS

EDMUND A. BERMUDEZ, MD, MPH, Assistant Professor of Medicine, Tufts University School of Medicine, Boston, Massachusetts; Department of Cardiovascular Medicine, Lahey Clinic, Burlington, Massachusetts

ROBERT O. BONOW, MD, Professor of Medicine and Chief, Division of Cardiology, Feinberg School of Medicine, Northwestern University, Chicago, Illinois

JEFFREY S. BORER, MD, Gladys and Roland Harriman Professor of Cardiovascular Medicine and Director, The Howard Gilman Institute for Valvular Heart Disease, Weill Medical College of Cornell University, New York, New York

ABRAHAM BORNSTEIN, MD, Assistant Professor of Medicine (formerly), Division of Cardiovascular Pathophysiology, The Howard Gilman Institute for Valvular Heart Diseases, Weill Medical College of Cornell University, New York Presbyterian Hospital, New York, New York

BLASE A. CARABELLO, MD, The W.A. "Tex," Jr, and Deborah Moncrief Professor of Medicine and Vice-Chairman, Department of Medicine, Baylor College of Medicine; Medical Care Line Executive, Veterans Affairs Medical Center, Houston, Texas

JOHN D. CARROLL, MD, Director and Professor of Medicine, University of Colorado Health Sciences, Denver, Colorado

JOHN N. CARTER, PhD, The Howard Gilman Institute of Valvular Heart Disease, Weill Medical College of Cornell University, New York, New York

DANIEL F. CATANZARO, PhD, The Howard Gilman Institute of Valvular Heart Disease, Weill Medical College of Cornell University, New York, New York

WILLIAM H. GAASCH, MD, Professor of Medicine, University of Massachusetts Medical School, Worcester, Massachusetts; Department of Cardiovascular Medicine, Lahey Clinic, Burlington, Massachusetts

EDMUND McM. HERROLD, MD, PhD, The Howard Gilman Institute of Valvular Heart Disease, Weill Medical College of Cornell University, New York, New York

GEU-RU HONG, MD, University of California Irvine, Orange, California

ANDREW J.P. KLEIN, MD, Fellow in Cardiovascular Disease, University of Colorado Health Sciences, Denver, Colorado

PENG LI, MD, PhD, University of California Irvine, Orange, California

JACEK PREIBISZ, MD, PhD, Adjunct Associate Professor of Medicine, Division of Cardiovascular Pathophysiology, The Howard Gilman Institute for Valvular Heart Diseases, Weill Medical College of Cornell University, New York Presbyterian Hospital, New York, New York

NALINI M. RAJAMANNAN, MD, FACC, FAHA, Valve Director, Bluhm Cardiovascular Institute, Northwestern Memorial Hospital; Department of Cardiology, Northwestern University Feinberg School of Medicine, Chicago, Illinois

VERA H. RIGOLIN, MD, Associate Professor of Medicine, Feinberg School of Medicine, Northwestern University, Chicago, Illinois

WILLIAM J. STEWART, MD, FACC, FASE, Associate Professor of Medicine, Cleveland Clinic Lerner College of Medicine; and Staff Cardiologist, Department of Cardiovascular Medicine, Section of Cardiovascular Imaging, The Cleveland Clinic Foundation, Cleveland, Ohio

PHYLLIS G. SUPINO, EdD, Associate Research Professor of Public Health in Medicine and Associate Research Professor of Public Health; and Director of Data Management, Epidemiology, and Educational Programs, Division of Cardiovascular Pathophysiology, The Howard Gilman Institute for Valvular Heart Diseases, Weill Medical College of Cornell University, New York Presbyterian Hospital, New York, New York

WALTER TSANG, MD, University of California Irvine, Orange, California

MANI A. VANNAN, MBBS, FACC, Professor of Medicine, University of California Irvine, Orange, California

CONTENTS

Valvular heart diseases (VHDs) are predictable causes of heart failure and significantly associated with sudden death. Doppler echocardiography enables detection and evaluation of VHD severity. Epidemiologic data defining prevalence and clinical correlates of VHDs from cross-sectional clinical series and population-based studies indicate that VHDs affect a large proportion of the population and that many persons manifest moderate or severe VHDs, even if clinically silent. Temporal trends in VHD diagnoses and surgical interventions from longitudinal studies show that echocardiographic and clinical diagnoses of VHDs and mechanical interventions to correct these disorders have increased markedly since the early 1980s. It is unclear whether these estimates are due to improved detection, to increasing disease prevalence, or both. Research and health care resources should be targeted toward meeting this public health challenge.

Calcific aortic stenosis is the most common indication for surgical valve replacement in the United States. This article reviews the pathogenesis and the potential for medical therapy in the management of patients who have this disease process. The author provides an overview of the emerging experimental and clinical studies important in the understanding of the cellular mechanisms of calcific aortic stenosis and addresses the growing number of retrospective and prospective clinical studies evaluating the use of statins as a potential for cholesterol-lowering treatment to prevent progression of aortic valve calcification.

Valvular heart diseases are disorders of the valvular structures that control blood flow into and out of the four cardiac chambers. When valves fail to open or close normally (ie, when they are stenotic or regurgitant), abnormal pressure or volume loads are imposed on the ventricular and atrial myocardium, leading to cellular and molecular adaptations that ultimately can result in heart failure and premature death. The authors' primary focus is the disordered biology of the cardiac fibroblast and extracellular matrix (ECM) in aortic regurgitation (AR) as an example of the knowledge emerging in the area of valvular diseases. Selected data relating to the cardiomyocyte in AR, aortic stenosis (AS), and mitral regurgitation (MR), and comparative information about the ECM in AS, is provided to emphasize the important differences among these diseases.

FORTHCOMING ISSUES

RECENT ISSUES

ELSEVIER
SAUNDERS

Heart Failure Clin 2 (2006) ix–x

HEART
FAILURE
CLINICS

Editorial
Mister Rogers' Neighborhood...

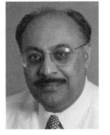 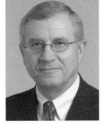

Jagat Narula, MD, PhD   James B. Young, MD
Consulting Editors

Continuing investigation is altering our perception of how and why valvular heart disease leads to ventricular remodeling and heart failure. For sometime now, a "hemodynamic" hypothesis ("load" and response to load) was used to explain this transition to heart failure. Knowledge of the altered loading conditions was necessary for the management of heart failure patients with valvular heart disease. Later, data brought prominence to the "neurohormonal" hypothesis, where secondary changes in local and circulating hormones played a role in the transition from clinical stability to manifest heart failure. Data now are starting to parse out cellular and molecular biodynamic changes during this transition, with many of these changes seem to predicating response to pharmacologic therapy. Clinicians, when planning treatment, do not incorporate alterations at cellular level into a therapeutic strategy. Future interventions might have to consider dynamic changes in the cardiomyocyte and interstitial components to fine-tune response to therapy. Recent data have elegantly clarified subcellular dissimilarities between pressure and volume overload cardiomyopathy of valvular heart disease and the potential influence on therapy [1,2].

Two major patterns of ventricular remodeling are described during the transition from injury to heart failure. Concentric remodeling, which is associated with pressure overload (eg, aortic stenosis, where increased myocardial mass is associated with normal left ventricular [LV] dimensions) and eccentric remodeling that is associated with volume overload (eg, mitral and aortic regurgitation, where increased myocardial mass is associated with an increased LV dimensions). The nature and duration of pressure and volume overload may differentially affect cardiomyocyte and interstitial remodeling. In pressure-overload states, increased systolic wall stress is associated with myocellular hypertrophy; subsequent development of interstitial fibrosis heralds functional deterioration. On the other hand, in volume overload states, increased diastolic wall stress is associated with lengthening of myocytes and loss (or minimal increase until late) of interstitial collagen, and contractile function remains relatively preserved. In both volume and pressure overload states, myocellular length to width ratio is initially preserved. Although a disproportionate increase in myocyte length accompanies decompensation, it is becoming clear that myocyte remodeling alone may not result in global dysfunction, and inhibiting myocyte remodeling may not always resolve functional deficit. This makes interstitial alteration an important candidate for therapeutic targeting. Importantly, angiotensin II is up-regulated prominently in valvular heart disease, and most of its receptors are located on the fibroblasts [3]. This would make angiotensin-converting enzyme (ACE) inhibitors the neurohumoral antagonist of choice. But very interestingly, there seems to be a discordance of their efficacy between pressure and volume overload; ACE inhibitors seem to be effective in pressure overload but largely ineffective in valvular regurgitation.

The reason why ACE inhibitor therapy is ineffective in the remodeling of volume overload is unclear but recent studies have proposed interesting concepts. Volume overload is associated with loss of interstitial collagen secondary to bradykinin-induced matrix metalloproteinase-mediated degradation. Since ACE inhibitors increase bradykinin, it is likely that ACE inhibitors may worsen this and thus be ineffective. However, bradykinin is also known to restrict ventricular remodeling in many conditions through its potent antigrowth influence that may predominantly attenuate fibrosis. Since ACE inhibitors have not been shown to worsen volume overload remodeling, it is logical to assume that they are beneficial only in conditions where there is significant fibrous tissue proliferation. As discussed and proposed recently [1], the benefits of ACE inhibitors in valvular heart disease seem to correlate less with cardiac or cardiomyocyte remodeling and more with extent of fibrosis. Thus, ACE inhibitors are useful in pressure overload (with significant interstitial fibrosis) but much less beneficial in volume overload (where there is minimal fibrosis). This concept is important, since noninvasive techniques of quantifying fibrosis are being developed and this therapy might influence therapeutic decisions [3]. It is now necessary that we pay attention to interstitial alterations, better understand the interactions of myocytes and interstitium, and learn to manipulate these components in isolation. An inordinate focus on the contracting cell may not be necessary and the importance of the interstitial

neighborhood of cardiomyocytes may not be underestimated. Indeed, Mister Rogers' neighborhood is, in the normal state, utopia. When perturbed, the neighborhood falls apart. We must better understand the pathophysiology or remodeling and development management algorithms accordingly.

Jagat Narula, MD, PhD
Professor, Medicine
Chief, Division of Cardiology
University of California
School of Medicine
101 The City Drive
Building 53, Mail Route 81
Orange, CA 92868, USA

E-mail address: narula@uci.edu

James B. Young, MD
Chairman, Department of Medicine
Professor, Medicine
Lerner College of Medicine
Case Western Reserve University
Cleveland Clinic Foundation
9500 Euclid Avenue
Desk T-13
Cleveland, OH 44195, USA

E-mail address: youngj@ccf.org

References

[1] Chandrashekhar Y. Embracing diversity in remodeling: a step in therapeutic decision making in heart failure. J Am Coll Cardiol 2007;49(7):822–5.
[2] Ryan TD, Rothstein EC, Immaculada A. LV eccentric remodeling and matrix loss are mediated by bradykinin and precede cardiomyocyte elongation in rats with volume over load. J Am Coll Cardiol 2007;49(7):811–21.
[3] Shirani J, Narula J, Eckelman WC, et al. Early imaging in heart failure: exploring novel molecular targets. J Nucl Cardiol 2007;14(1):100–10.

ELSEVIER
SAUNDERS

Heart Failure Clin 2 (2006) xi

HEART
FAILURE
CLINICS

Preface

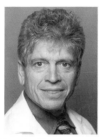

Blase A. Carabello, MD
Guest Editor

This issue of the *Heart Failure Clinics* emphasizes the role of valvular heart disease (VHD) as a cause of heart failure. Though not as prevalent as coronary disease or primary muscle disease in causing the syndrome, VHD is important for at least three major reasons.

First, VHDs are diseases of aging. The impact of valve disease increases as the population gets older, which is emphasized well in the article by Supino and colleagues.

Second, unlike coronary disease and dilated cardiomyopathy, heart failure caused by VHD can be reversed entirely when the valve abnormalities are corrected with proper timing. Thus, the understanding of the pathophysiology of VHD and the proper timing of intervention can rid the patient who has heart failure from VHD permanently. These topics are discussed in the articles by Rigolin and Bonow, Klein and Carroll, Bermudez and Gaasch, and Stewart.

Third, we are beginning to understand the mechanisms of VHD, pertaining to the causes of the valve abnormalities themselves (see the article by Rajamannan) and the molecular mechanisms of ventricular damage (see the articles by Carabello and Borer and colleagues).

The contributions to this issue by leading experts in the field are timely and cutting edge and should provide the reader with knowledge helpful both in the clinic and in the basic laboratory. We hope readers find this issue informative, easy to read, and useful in treating VHD.

Blase A. Carabello, MD
Department of Medicine
Baylor College of Medicine
One Baylor Plaza
Houston, TX, USA

Veterans Affairs Medical Center
2002 Holcombe Blvd
Houston, TX 77030, USA

E-mail address:
blaseanthony.carabello@med.va.gov

1551-7136/06/$ - see front matter © 2007 Elsevier Inc. All rights reserved.
doi:10.1016/j.hfc.2007.02.003

ELSEVIER
SAUNDERS

Heart Failure Clin 2 (2006) 379–393

HEART
FAILURE
CLINICS

The Epidemiology of Valvular Heart Disease: a Growing Public Health Problem

Phyllis G. Supino, EdD*, Jeffrey S. Borer, MD,
Jacek Preibisz, MD, PhD, Abraham Bornstein, MD

Weill Medical College of Cornell University, New York Presbyterian Hospital, New York, NY, USA

Valvular heart diseases (VHDs), as a group, are among the most predictable causes of heart failure (HF) [1]. They are also potentially lethal, particularly among patients who have been conservatively managed [2,3] because sudden death in patients who have VHDs is relatively common, even in the absence of other risk factors [3]. Recent data compiled by the American Heart Association indicate that mortality due to VHDs in the United States is approximately 20,000 patients annually [4] or about 7 per 100,000 population. Although the aortic and mitral valves are most frequently implicated, the tricuspid and pulmonic

valves can also be dysfunctional, leading to adverse outcomes.

Before the use of Doppler echocardiography, the prevalence of VHDs was poorly defined and generally underestimated. In the current era characterized by frequent noninvasive imaging and informed by cross-sectional and longitudinal studies, it is clear that a remarkably high proportion of the population has asymptomatic VHD [5–7]. These studies suggest that asymptomatic VHD generally progresses slowly from hemodynamically mild to relative hemodynamic severity, after which a relatively prolonged "latent period" ensues until clinical debility or death [8]. Moreover, at least in the United States and Western Europe, the etiology of VHDs is now largely degenerative or idiopathic [9,10] (probably based at least in part on specific genetic predispositions). This etiology represents an important change from the predominance 50 or more years ago of rheumatic (postinfectious) causation [11]. Therefore, because expression of VHD now most often occurs after the age of procreation, the total number of affected persons will increase as the population ages and grows. As intercurrent causes of death and debility are increasingly eradicated, and as therapeutic options are developed and perfected, this population increasingly becomes a target for interventions that prolong life and improve its quality. This article reviews available epidemiologic data about prevalence and clinical correlates of eight forms of VHD from published cross-sectional clinical series and population-based studies from several countries, and examines temporal trends in VHD diagnoses and

Dr. Borer was supported in part during this work by an endowment from The Gladys and Roland Harriman Foundation. This work also was supported by grants from The Howard Gilman Foundation, The Schiavone Family Foundation, The Charles and Jean Brunie Foundation, The David Margolis Foundation, The American Cardiovascular Research Foundation, The Irving A. Hansen Foundation, The Mary A.H. Rumsey Foundation, The Messinger Family Foundation, The Daniel and Elaine Sargent Charitable Trust, The A.C. Israel Foundation, and by much appreciated gifts from Donna and William Acquavella, Maryjane Voute Arrigoni, the late William Voute, Gerald Tanenbaum, and Stephen and Suzanne Weiss.

* Corresponding author. Division of Cardiovascular Pathophysiology, The Howard Gilman Institute for Valvular Heart Diseases, Weill Medical College of Cornell University, New York Presbyterian Hospital, 525 E. 68th Street, Room F467, New York, NY 10021.

E-mail address: phs2002@med.cornell.edu (P.G. Supino).

surgical interventions from longitudinal studies conducted in the United States.

Prevalence of pure, isolated valve diseases

Aortic stenosis

Among valve lesions that are recognized as hemodynamically severe and that receive clinical attention, aortic stenosis (AS) is the most common in the United States; this lesion clearly increases in prevalence and severity with advancing age [12]. AS usually results from fibrosis and calcification of the aortic leaflets of trileaflet aortic valves; however, although far less frequently expressed than trileaflet valves, congenitally bicuspid aortic valves (a variant present in 1%–2% of the population [13]) are more likely to calcify and to become stenotic than trileaflet valves. In asymptomatic patients who have severe AS, life expectancy is nearly normal until syncope, angina, or HF supervene; the 5-year survival rate is estimated to be 50% or less after symptoms develop, an expectation that can be further modified by left ventricular (LV) geometric and hemodynamic characteristics and exercise capacity [14,15].

AS prevalence has been evaluated specifically among patients older than 60 years by Aronow and colleagues [16] who applied M-mode, two-dimensional (2-D), continuous wave Doppler, and pulsed Doppler echocardiography in 1797 residents of a long-term health care facility. AS prevalence was similar in men (14%) and women

(18%) (Table 1). Among women, AS was mild in 10%, moderate in 6%, and severe in 2% [17]; among men, severity was not reported, and the relation of AS prevalence/severity to age or other clinical factors within the older-than-60-years cohort was not evaluated. Subsequently, prevalence of AS in relation to age was reported from the Helsinki Ageing Study, which evaluated 552 randomly selected men and women subgrouped according to age (55–71, 75–76, 80–81, and 85–86 years) [18]. All subjects underwent echocardiography (M-mode, 2-D, and continuous wave, pulsed, and color Doppler). AS was found only in the three older age groups and increased with advancing age (Table 2); the prevalence of moderate AS among these patients was 4.8%; "critically" severe AS was found in 2.9%. No differences in prevalence were noted with regard to sex or other clinical factors [18]. Finally, the largest population-based study of AS prevalence was conducted in the United States among 5201 men and women 65 years and older who were enrolled in the Cardiovascular Health Study, a prospective longitudinal study including comprehensive clinical and echocardiographic (2-D and continuous wave Doppler) data [19]. Although one in four subjects had structurally apparent valve deformity ("visually apparent" leaflet thickening, calcification, or both [19]), the prevalence of hemodynamically definable AS (severity not reported) was 1.5% among women and 2.0% among men and, consistent with findings from the Helsinki Ageing Study, rose with advancing age (Table 3). Other factors

Table 1
Prevalence of echocardiographic findings in older men and women

Variable	Men (n = 554)	Women (n = 1243)	P
Rheumatic mitral stenosis	2 (0.4)	20 (2)	.034
Mitral annular calcium	194 (35)	665 (53)	<.0001
≥1 + Mitral regurgitation	176 (32)	415 (33)	NS
Aortic stenosis	79 (14)	222 (18)	NS
≥1 + Aortic regurgitation	174 (31)	352 (28)	NS
Hypertrophic cardiomyopathy	15 (3)	47 (4)	NS
Idiopathic dilated cardiomyopathy	6 (1)	10 (1)	NS
Left atrial enlargement	159 (29)	460 (37)	.001
LV hypertrophy	226 (41)	539 (43)	NS
Abnormal LV ejection fraction	159 (29)	263 (21)	.0006

Data are expressed as number (%) of subjects.
Abbreviation: NS, not significant.
Data from Aronow WS, Ahn C, Kronzon I. Prevalence of echocardiographic findings in 554 men and 1,243 women aged >60 years in a long-term health facility. Am J Cardiol 1997;79(3):379–80.

Table 2
Frequency of aortic valve stenosis in the different age groups based on the combined criteria of velocity ratio ≥0.35 and calculated aortic valve area (the Helsinki Ageing Study)

Aortic valve area (cm^2)	Age group (y)		
	75–76[a] (n = 197)	80–81 (n = 155)	85–86 (n = 124)
≤1.2	5 (2.5)	6 (3.9)	10 (8.1)
≤1.0	4 (2.0)	4 (2.6)	10 (8.1)
≤0.8	1 (0.5)	4 (2.6)	10 (8.1)
≤0.6	0 (0.0)	3 (1.9)	4 (3.2)
≤0.4	0 (0.0)	0 (0.0)	1 (0.8)

The data are given as the number of persons (% of age group) in each age and valve area category. The increase in the prevalence of aortic stenosis with age is statistically significant (P = .05). No case of aortic valve stenosis was detected among the 76 patients aged 55–71 years.

[a] Two persons in this age group had an aortic valve prosthesis; they are not included in the frequency data.

Data from Lindroos M, Kupari M, Heikkila J, et al. Prevalence of aortic valve abnormalities in the elderly: an echocardiographic study of a random population sample. J Am Coll Cardiol 1993;21(5):1220–5.

associated with AS (or with aortic sclerosis) in this population included male sex, lipoproteins Lp(a) and LDL cholesterol, height, history of hypertension, and current smoking [19]. Taken together, these data suggest that hemodynamically severe AS is present in at least 2% of persons older than 70 years.

Aortic regurgitation

Aortic regurgitation (AR) can result from aortic leaflet abnormalities including congenitally bicuspid aortic valve and deformities caused by infective endocarditis or rheumatic fever (RF); from aortic root dilatation associated with hypertension, aging, aortic dissection, bicuspid aortic valve, Marfan syndrome, or other connective tissue variants or collagen vascular diseases; and from other, currently less common etiologies like syphilis [20]. The natural history of chronic AR is characterized by a long asymptomatic interval, even when AR is severe. In most patients, LV dysfunction ultimately occurs (with or without symptoms) and leads to death unless surgery is performed [21]. Among asymptomatic patients who have severe AR and normal LV ejection fraction at rest, progression to subnormal LV ejection fraction, overt HF, or death occurs at a rate of 4% to 6% per year [10,22,23]. In acute AR (most commonly caused by endocarditis and less

Table 3
Prevalence of aortic valve abnormalities by echocardiography (the Cardiovascular Health Study)

Subjects	Aortic valve abnormality			
	None	Sclerosis	Stenosis	Valve replacement
All subjects	3736 (72)	1329 (26)	88 (2)	23 (0.4)
Women	2249 (76)	641 (22)	43 (1.5)	12 (0.4)
Men	1487 (67)	688 (31)	45 (2)	11 (0.5)
65–74 y	2684 (78)	697 (20)	43 (1.3)	16 (0.5)
Women	1654 (82)	344 (17)	20 (1.0)	9 (0.4)
Men	1030 (73)	353 (25)	23 (1.6)	7 (0.5)
75–84 y	962 (62)	542 (35)	37 (2.4)	7 (0.5)
Women	546 (66)	259 (31)	22 (2.7)	3 (0.4)
Men	416 (58)	283 (39)	15 (2.1)	4 (0.6)
85+ y	90 (48)	90 (48)	8 (4)	0 (0)
Women	49 (56)	38 (43)	1 (1)	0 (0)
Men	41 (41)	52 (52)	7 (7)	0 (0)

Data are expressed as number (%) of subjects.
Data from Stewart B, Siscovick D, Lind BK. Clinical factors associated with calcific aortic valve disease. J Am Coll Cardiol 1997;29(3):630–34.

commonly by aortic dissection), the sudden increase in LV filling can result in the rapid onset of HF or death unless surgical intervention is performed quickly [24].

Early studies of AR prevalence involved relatively small groups of normal volunteers or patients of differing ages who had undergone pulsed or continuous wave Doppler echocardiographic assessment [25–32]. These studies produced widely varying estimates, ranging from 0% in one study of children (0–14 years old, n = 461) who had "structurally normal" hearts assessed by 2-D echocardiography [31] and in another study of apparently healthy volunteers (6–49 years old, n = 211) [27], to 39% in a study of older subjects (40–90 years old, n = 176) [26] (Table 4). In all cases, AR severity was described as trivial or mild. More recently, large population-based observational studies using color Doppler echocardiography have suggested a different pattern. One of the first studies, the Coronary Artery Risk Development in Young Adults (CARDIA) sponsored by the National Heart, Lung, and Blood Institute (NHLBI) estimated the prevalence and clinical correlates of AR (and mitral regurgitation [MR]) in a multicenter study of free-living men and women (23–35 years old, n = 4352) originally recruited from 1985 to 1986 [5]. AR was found in 1.2% (mild in 79%) and was unrelated to sex (1.4% of men versus 1.0% of women) or to race (1.1% of blacks versus 1.3% of whites) [5]. A subsequent study of 3589 unselected men and women (54 ± 10 years old) who had undergone color Doppler echocardiography between 1991 and 1995 was reported from the NHLBI-sponsored Framingham Heart Study. AR of trace-or-greater severity was found in 13.0% of men and 8.5% of women; the clinical correlates of AR were advancing age and, unlike the findings from CARDIA, male sex (Table 5) [6]. AR prevalence was also recently evaluated in the second NHLBI-sponsored Strong Heart Study of 3501 men and women (46–82 years old; mean, 60 years) from 13 United States American Indian tribes; this cohort included a relatively high proportion of middle- to older-age, overweight persons [33]. M-mode, 2-D, and pulsed, continuous wave, and color Doppler echocardiography were employed in all subjects. AR was found in 10% of subjects (mild [1+] in 7.3%, moderate [2+] in 2.4%, and moderately severe to severe [3–4+] in 0.3%) and was independently and directly

Table 4
Prevalence of valvular regurgitation in normal subjects: results of Doppler echocardiographic surveys

Study	Population	Prevalence[a](%)			
		AR	MR	TR	PR
Kostucki et al, 1986 [25]	25 normal subjects aged 15–18 y	33	40	40	92
Akasaka et al, 1987 [26]	176 healthy volunteers aged 40–90 y	39	34	39	30
Yoshida et al, 1988 [27]	211 healthy volunteers aged 6–49 y	0	42	52	57
Berger et al, 1989 [28]	100 healthy volunteers aged 23–89 y	1	21	50	31
Choong et al, 1989 [29]	867 patients, structurally normal hearts[b], from birth to >80 y	3	19	17	5
Klein et al, 1990 [30]	118 healthy volunteers[b] aged 21–82 y	11	48	65	31
Brand et al, 1992 [31]	461 patients, structurally normal hearts[b], from birth to 14 y	0	2	6	22
Lavie et al, 1993 [32]	206 patients, structurally normal hearts[b], aged 15–86 y	12	73	68	NA

Abbreviations: A, aortic; M, mitral; NA, not available; P, pulmonary; R, regurgitation; T, tricuspid.
[a] Trace on more regurgitation (rates rounded).
[b] By 2-D echocardiography.

Table 5
Valvular regurgitation prevalence in the Framingham Heart Study by age, sex, and severity

Severity	Age									
	26–39 y		40–49 y		50–59 y		60–69 y		70–83 y	
	M	W	M	W	M	W	M	W	M	W
AR severity										
None	96.7	98.9	95.4	96.6	91.1	92.4	74.3	86.9	75.6	73.0
Trace	3.3	1.1	2.9	2.7	4.7	5.5	13.0	6.3	10.0	10.1
Mild	0.0	0.0	1.4	0.7	3.7	1.9	12.1	6.0	12.2	14.6
Moderate or greater	0.0	0.0	0.3	0.0	0.5	0.2	0.6	0.8	2.2	2.3
MR severity										
None	14.4	14.0	13.3	8.6	11.3	9.0	12.7	7.2	9.0	5.6
Trace	76.7	76.3	72.9	75.0	74.6	74.0	60.3	66.5	51.7	70.8
Mild	8.9	9.7	13.5	15.5	12.5	16.0	24.6	24.0	28.1	23.6
Moderate or greater	0.0	0.0	0.3	0.9	1.6	1.0	2.4	2.3	11.2	0.0
TR severity										
None	14.3	20.5	17.8	16.0	19.0	14.5	18.3	10.4	16.7	14.1
Trace	72.7	65.1	72.5	70.0	71.5	70.7	59.8	62.2	47.0	56.4
Mild	13.0	13.2	9.4	13.5	9.2	14.1	21.9	25.7	25.8	23.9
Moderate or greater	0.0	1.2	0.3	0.5	0.3	0.7	0.0	1.7	1.5	5.6

Data are presented as percentage of subjects (N = 3589; 1696 men, 1893 women).

Abbreviations: M, men; MR, mitral regurgitation; TR, tricuspid regurgitation; W, women.

Data from Singh JP, Evans JC, Levy D, et al. Prevalence and clinical determinants of mitral, tricuspid and aortic regurgitation (the Framingham Heart Study). Am J Cardiol 1999;83(6):897–902.

associated with age (Fig. 1), aortic root diameter, aortic and mitral stenosis (MS), absence of diabetes, and albuminuria but not with sex, body mass index (BMI), height, or hypertension [33].

Mitral stenosis

MS is usually a consequence of RF [34] contracted during childhood or adolescence but

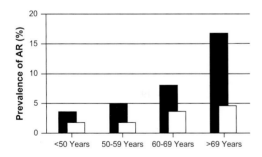

Fig. 1. The prevalence of mild (1+) AR (*solid bars*) and more severe (≥2+) AR (*open bars*) in Strong Heart Study participants shows strong positive correlations to increasing age (*P* < .001). (*From* Lebowitz NE, Bella JN, Roman MJ, et al. Prevalence and correlates of aortic regurgitation in American Indians: the Strong Heart Study. J Am Coll Cardiol 2000;36:463; with permission. Copyright 2000, American College of Cardiology Foundation.)

occasionally occurs congenitally or as a result of degenerative disease with annular calcification among adults. An unusual but recognized cause of MS and of other valve diseases is radiation-induced injury [35] among patients who have received chest radiation for Hodgkin's disease or other cancers. Following an initial asymptomatic period (of up to 20 years), most patients will develop HF of increasing severity over time [36]. Approximately one fourth of all patients who have RF develop pure MS and another 40% develop combined MS and MR [37]. In developing countries where repeated occurrences of RF are common, severe MS may become clinically manifest within 2 to 5 years of an episode of RF and is independent of sex [38]; this form of MS is referred to as "juvenile MS." In the United States or in other developed countries, however, MS typically occurs decades after acute RF, affecting women two to three times more frequently than men [39]. Although once widespread in the United States (100–200 cases per 100,000 population at the turn of the twentieth century) [40], RF has steadily declined (despite scattered focal areas of resurgence in the mid- to late-1980s [41–46]) to approximately 2 cases per 100,000 population in the 1990s (Fig. 2) [41], resulting in a concomitant decline in MS [39]. A parallel decline in rheumatic MS has been documented in Europe [47].

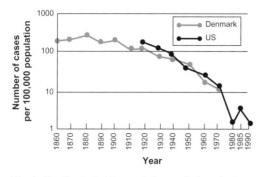

Fig. 2. Decline in incidence of rheumatic fever in Denmark and United States. (*From* Ayoub EM. Resurgence of rheumatic fever in the United States. The changing picture of a preventable illness. Postgrad Med 1992; 92(3):134; with permission. Copyright 1992, Vendome Group LLC.)

Available data from the United States, Canada, Europe, and Japan, compiled in the 1970s and 1980s, revealed a mean age for diagnosis of MS of 50 to 60 years, in sharp contrast to China, Saudi Arabia, India, Korea, and South Africa, where mean of age at diagnosis ranged between 20 and 39 years [38]. Accordingly, in the 1990s in the United States, MS was labeled a "geriatric disease" [48], albeit of low prevalence. Thus, in Aronow and colleagues' [16] 1997 study of nursing home residents older than 60 years (to the authors' knowledge, the sole peer-reviewed report of MS prevalence in any Western adult population), MS of "rheumatic origin" was present in 0.4% of men and 2% of women (see Table 1). Because these data do not include new cases among young people or account for trends in immigration and, thus, may not be sensitive to the changing demographics of the United States [38], they possibly underestimate the current prevalence of MS in this country. It is unfortunate that more recent population-based assessments of MS prevalence, including increasing numbers of young immigrants to this country since the late 1980s from areas where rheumatic heart disease is common (eg, Mexico, Central and South America, and Asia), are not currently available.

Mitral regurgitation

MR most commonly results from the leaflet/chordal variations of mitral valve prolapse (due to "myxomatous degeneration" or other genetically determined factors) or from myocardial ischemia (due to coronary artery disease with or without prior myocardial infarction), with loss of normal valvular support or other geometric deformity. MR also can result from infective endocarditis, collagen vascular disease, ruptured chordae tendineae of various etiologies, or from RF [20]. In asymptomatic subjects who have chronic severe MR, the clinical course progresses with moderate rapidity (and more rapidly than AR); the average risk of developing HF or worse is approximately 10% per year if surgery is not performed [49,50]. Acute MR (usually caused by an ischemic event or by endocarditis, although acute flail leaflet due to chordal rupture can also result from mitral valve prolapse or other etiologies) has a significantly poorer prognosis; surgical mortality is relatively high when ischemia or endocarditis is the cause [51]. In contrast to MS, prevalence of MR has been well characterized by echocardiographic and population-based studies, although ischemic versus nonischemic etiologies are not typically differentiated in these studies. As for AR, early studies of MR prevalence involved normal volunteers or patients who had undergone Doppler echocardiography [25–32]. Again, as in AR, these studies produced discrepant estimates of MR prevalence (trivial or mild), ranging from 2.4% [31] to 73% [32] (see Table 4); several of these estimates varied directly with age [26,28–30]. Among later studies that were population based, prevalence of MR of at least mild severity ranged from 11% (CARDIA study [5]) to 19% and 21%, respectively (Framingham Heart Study [6] and Strong Heart Study [7]), rates that were markedly higher than those found for AR in the same populations. MR prevalence in CARDIA was similar among men (11.2%) and women (10.7%) and among blacks (11.0) and whites (10.9%) [5]. No severe MR was documented in this relatively young (23–35 years) population [52] and no associations with age were reported. MR was detected in 87.7% of men (19.0% mild-or-greater severity) and 91.5% of women (19.1% mild-or-greater severity) in the Framingham Heart Study involving an older population [6]. Strong associations were shown between MR of mild-or-greater severity and advancing age (see Table 5); when analyzed according to degree of severity, the prevalence of mild (1+) and of moderate-to-severe (≥2+) MR increased by decade of age. Other clinical correlates were (lower) BMI, HF, myocardial infarction, and systemic hypertension [6]. In the Strong Heart Study, mild (1+) MR was found in 19.2%, moderate (2+) MR in 1.6%, moderately severe (3+) MR in 0.3%, and severe (4+) MR in 0.2% [7]. As in the Framingham Heart

Study, MR prevalence was independently associated with age (Fig. 3) and lower BMI; unlike the Framingham Heart Study, the presence (but not severity) of MR was associated with female sex but not with hypertension [7]. Other independent correlates of MR defined by the Strong Heart Study included higher serum creatinine, lower BMI, associated MS, prior myocardial infarction, and mitral valve prolapse [7].

Tricuspid stenosis

Tricuspid stenosis (TS) results from structural alterations of the tricuspid valve leaflets that impede excursion, thereby obstructing right atrial emptying into the right ventricle and pulmonary vasculature. TS is almost always of rheumatic origin and usually occurs among patients who have MS or other acquired valvular diseases but may also result from congenital anomalies, right atrial tumors, or carcinoid syndrome [36]. When uncorrected, over time, TS may result in venous engorgement, invariably producing edema, ascites, and hepatomegaly [53]. Operative mortality (generally high) is related to preoperative functional class, severity of HF, and magnitude of chronic hemodynamic changes in the right atrium and pulmonary circulation [54]. The first studies to estimate TS prevalence were based on necropsy or clinical series of patients who had rheumatic heart disease and conducted outside the United States. The earliest of the necropsy studies, conducted between the 1920s and 1950s (meta-analyzed by Kitchin and Turner [55]), produced rates that varied widely (22%–44%) and were

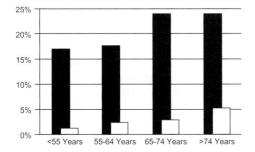

Fig. 3. The prevalence (%) of mild (1+) MR (*black bars*) increased by decade of age as did that of 2+ or greater MR (*white bars*) (*P* < .001). (*From* Jones EC, Devereux RB, Roman MJ, et al. Prevalence and correlates of mitral regurgitation in a population-based sample (the Strong Heart Study). Am J Cardiol 2001;87(3): 300; with permission. Copyright 2001, Excerpta Medica, Inc.)

higher than rates (14%) found by these investigators in a necropsy study at their own institution in the 1960s [55]. Clinical studies conducted during the same period among patients undergoing surgery for severe MS indicated lower TS prevalence, ranging from 3%–15% [55,56]. More recent echocardiographic surveys, conducted among patients who had RF in India, have also reported relatively low TS rates (4.4% [TS ± other VHDs] [57]; 0.5%–0.6% [isolated] [57,58]). Disparities in these prevalence rates are arguably due to variations in diagnostic criteria and modality (visual inspection [necropsy] versus cardiac catheterization or echocardiography), differences in study group characteristics (living versus deceased patients, the latter probably heavily confounded by selection biases; medically managed versus surgical patients; isolated versus associated disease), and temporal and geographic factors. Like rheumatic mitral valve disease, TS has been observed more commonly in women than in men [53].

Tricuspid regurgitation

Tricuspid regurgitation (TR) may be caused by structural damage to valve leaflets due to RF [59], to other structural variants (including congenital anomalies—most commonly Ebstein's anomaly), and primarily in adults, to endocarditis, tricuspid valve prolapse, papillary muscle dysfunction (often ischemic), trauma, rheumatoid arthritis, and carcinoid syndrome [36]. More frequently, however, TR is "functional," meaning that it occurs as a result of stretching of the tricuspid annulus in association with right ventricle geometric alteration [60] that usually is caused by pulmonary hypertension (primary or secondary to left heart diseases). During the past decade, several cases of TR (usually with coexisting AR and MR) have also been reported among patients (primarily women) who were exposed to the appetite suppressants fenfluramine, or phentermine [61,62]. Mortality and morbidity associated with TR is directly related to the underlying cause [53] and severity [63]. Doppler echocardiographic surveys, conducted with 2-D echocardiography among apparently healthy volunteers or among patients who had presumably "structurally normal" hearts, have found high prevalence of TR (predominantly trace or mild), ranging from 17% in one study of 867 subjects (0 to >80 years old) with structurally normal hearts by 2-D echocardiography [29] to 68% in another study of 206 subjects who also had structurally normal hearts (15–86 years old; see Table 4) [32]. TR prevalence or severity was associated with advancing age in four of these eight studies [26,29,30,32] and with female sex in two [28,29]. TR (any severity) was detectable in 82.0% of men and 85.7% of women in the Framingham Heart Study—to the authors' knowledge, the only truly population-based study to quantify this form of VHD. TR prevalence of mild-or-greater and moderate-or-greater severity was found in 14.8% and 0.3% of men, respectively, and in 18.4% and 1.2% of women, respectively, in this population [6]. Clinical determinants of TR were advancing age, lower BMI, and female sex [6]. When analyzed across successive age groupings, TR of mild-or-greater severity increased with advancing age among men and women (see Table 5) and, as in MR, was negatively correlated with BMI [6]. An unusual cause of TR seems to be cardiac transplantation: in several transplantation series, high incidences of TR, often mild, have been reported, ranging from 20% [64] to 78% [65]. In addition, a variable number of recipients develop severe TR after cardiac transplantation (ranging from 2.5% in 1 study [n = 336] [64] to 25% in another [n = 101] [66]) that has occasionally warranted surgical relief. The etiology of TR in this select population has been attributed to implantation technique, mismatch between donor and recipient heart size, infection, ischemic injury, and damage from repeated surveillance endocardial biopsy [64,66].

Pulmonary stenosis

Pulmonary stenosis (PS) is a hemodynamic obstruction of the right ventricular outflow tract, most commonly occurring at the level of the pulmonic valve. Valvular stenosis, the most common form (found in approximately 80%–90% of all PS) [67], is most often an isolated lesion but can also be found in association with other cardiac anomalies [68]. The usual presentation of PS is congenital. The clinical course during adulthood is largely benign, with little progression of stenosis [69]. Two epidemiologic reports published in the United States between 1980 and 1985 defined PS prevalence in two large pediatric populations. The New England Regional Infant Study (based on 1,528,686 live-born children in six New England states) found PS in 0.073/1000 live births, whereas the Baltimore-Washington Infant Study (based on 179,697 resident births in Maryland and the Washington, DC, metropolitan area) found PS in 0.189/1000 live births [70]. In

a large European study comprising 91,823 live-born children in Bohemia, PS was found in 7.13% of children who had documented congenital heart defects, or approximately 0.5/1000 live births [71]. A more recent (1998) study from Malta found a modestly higher prevalence of PS (1.65/1000 live births) during 1990 to 1994 [72], which was influenced perhaps at least in part by the increasing use of Doppler echocardiography to establish this diagnosis. To the authors' knowledge, there are no studies of PS prevalence among the general population of adults.

Pulmonary regurgitation

Pulmonary regurgitation (PR) may be congenital but is most commonly caused by dilation of the pulmonary valve ring due to primary or secondary pulmonary hypertension, although other etiologic substrates for this dilatation may be present [36]. Other causes of PR include complications of surgical repair of PS or other congenital heart diseases (most particularly tetralogy of Fallot [73]), sequelae of balloon catheter dilatation for PS [74], infective endocarditis [75], rheumatic heart disease [76], carcinoid heart disease [77], and Marfan syndrome [78]. Acquired PR is seldom hemodynamically important; however, over time, PR may adversely affect right ventricular function, leading to arrhythmia and sudden cardiac death [74]. The prevalence of PR (typically of trace-to-mild severity) has been detected in Doppler echocardiographic assessments among 5% to 92% of healthy volunteers or patients who had structurally normal hearts (see Table 4) in whom PR has been described as a normal physiologic variant. In most "normals," PR prevalence increased with advancing age (Fig. 4) [26,30,31], although in one study, a directionally opposite association was found [27] and, in two others [28,29], there was no association. As for AR, MR, and TR, variability of these estimates is undoubtedly due to differences in techniques, population characteristics, and sample sizes. The prevalence and severity of PR in the general population or among subsets who have cardiopulmonary diseases in which PR may be clinically important is not well defined, except among patients who have undergone surgical or percutaneous interventions involving the pulmonic valve (eg, for PS or tetralogy of Fallot repair). In such patients, prevalence of clinically important (ie, severe) PR has been in observed in 31%, increasing with postrepair age [79].

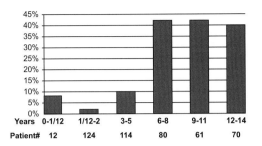

Fig. 4. Prevalence of PR stratified according to age. Prevalence increased significantly with age (*P* < .0001). The number of children who had normal hearts evaluated for presence of PR is indicated for each age group. (*From* Brand A, Dollberg S, Keren A. The prevalence of valvular regurgitation in children with structurally normal hearts: a color Doppler echocardiographic study. Am Heart J 1992;123(1):178; with permission. Copyright 1992, Elsevier, Inc.)

Relation of age and valvular heart diseases

As can be inferred from the aforementioned prevalence data, age is an important risk factor for valve disease. The authors have recently shown that the average age of patients who have this disorder has increased linearly over the past 2 decades [80]. In addition to these overall prevalence data, several Doppler echocardiographic studies of "normal" subjects have sought to characterize the number of regurgitant valves and the severity of regurgitation in the same individual in relation to advancing age [26,28–30,32]. In a study of 100 healthy volunteers (mean age, 45 ± 16 years) free of history/symptoms of cardiac disease, Berger and colleagues [28] detected regurgitation of one, two, or three valves (aortic, mitral, and tricuspid or pulmonic) in 46%, 24%, and 3%, respectively. No association was found between number of regurgitant lesions and age of the subject in this relatively young population. Similarly, in a study of 206 referred patients (mean age, 47 ± 4 years) who had completely normal M-mode or 2-D echocardiograms, Lavie and colleagues [32] found aortic, mitral, or TR (mild to moderate) of one valve in 38%, of two valves in 48%, and of three valves in 8%. As in Berger and colleagues' [28] study, multivalvular disease was not more common among older (>50 years) versus younger patients (≤50 years), although severity of MR and TR was age dependent [32]. In contrast, a strong and direct association between number of regurgitant valves (aortic, mitral, tricuspid, or pulmonic) and age was identified by Akasaka and colleagues [26] in a study of 176 volunteers (66 ± 14 years old) who had no history or physical evidence of cardiac abnormality (Table 6). Multivalvular regurgitation (predominantly trivial to mild but occasionally moderate) was noted among 51% of subjects 50 years or older and was common (89%) among those older than 80 years [26]. Akasaka and colleagues' [26] findings were confirmed by Choong and coworkers [29] in a study of Doppler findings in 867 patients (birth to ≥60 years) with normal 2-D echocardiograms and by Klein and colleagues [30] in a Doppler study of 118 apparently healthy volunteers (48 ± 17 years old) who also evaluated all four valves. The apparent discrepancies among these studies may be due to differences in sample size (most were relatively small) and age of the subjects; Doppler techniques; and definitions of regurgitation, statistical approaches, nature of the valves considered (ie, inclusion or exclusion of the pulmonic

Table 6
Number of regurgitant valves by age group: a Doppler study of "healthy" volunteers

	Age				
	40–49 y (n = 33)	50–59 y (n = 35)	60–69 y (n = 36)	70–79 y (n = 37)	80+ y (n = 35)
No. of regurgitant valves					
None	97	86	31	5	0
One	1	11	33	19	11
Two	0	3	25	22	23
Three	0	0	11	30	34
Four	0	0	0	24	31

Data are presented as percentage of subjects.
Data from Akasaka T, Yoshikawa J, Yoshida K, et al. Age-related valvular regurgitation: a study by pulsed Doppler echocardiography. Circulation 1987;76(2):262–5.

valve), and patient referral or subject recruitment patterns. The only true population-based study to evaluate number of regurgitant valves (the Framingham Heart Study) found regurgitation (mild-or-greater severity for mitral and tricuspid valves; trace-or-greater severity for aortic valve) of one, two, and three valves in approximately 25%, 9%, and less than 2%, respectively [6]; PR was not included in these estimates. Although prevalence and severity of AR, MR, and TR each increased with advancing age among men and women, the association of age and number of regurgitant valves per se was not evaluated in this study [6].

Temporal trends in valvular heart disease frequency

Only three studies have evaluated temporal trends in VHD prevalence in large populations. The first of these, a study by Ballard and colleagues [81], analyzed records from 95,745 echocardiograms performed by the Mayo Clinic between 1975 and 1986. More than 91% of these echocardiograms involved patients from outside Olmsted County, Minnesota (referral patients); the balance involved Olmsted County residents (a population-based cohort). These data revealed a marked increase in echocardiographic diagnoses of AR and MR (but not of biscuspid aortic valve or mitral valve prolapse) after 1982 (Table 7),

which coincided with the introduction of Doppler echocardiography at that facility in 1982 and its widespread use after 1984 [81]. Data pertaining to diagnostic indication for echocardiographic assessment, AR/MR severity, demographics, and outcomes were not available, limiting interpretability of these findings.

To obtain quantitative data for their region about clinical diagnoses and to provide new knowledge about the impact of VHD on the use of health care resources, the authors recently undertook a longitudinal study of VHD hospitalizations of more than 1 million patients hospitalized during an 18-year interval in New York State (1983–2000) [82]. The objectives of this study were to examine temporal trends in hospitalization rates and rates of surgery or other invasive therapeutic procedures among in-patients who had diagnoses of aortic, mitral, tricuspid, or pulmonic VHD, and to evaluate hospital mortality among patients who had these diseases. The source of data for this study was the New York Statewide Planning and Research Cooperative System (SPARCS) in-patient database, a comprehensive, computer-based information system developed by the New York State Department of Health to assist hospitals, government agencies, and health care organizations with decision making [83]. SPARCS comprises information for each discharge from the more than 250 nonfederal acute care facilities in 57 counties in New York State. Among the variables that are tabulated in SPARCS

Table 7
Temporal changes in echocardiographic diagnosis of valvular heart disease and disorders among residents of Olmsted County, Minnesota: 1975–1987

Year	% AR	% MR	% Biscupid AV	% MV prolapse
1975	4	9	<1	9
1976	8	6	2	10
1977	7	6	3	10
1978	4	3	3	12
1979	5	3	2	13
1980	4	3	3	12
1981	4	1	2	14
1982	4	2	2	12
1983	7	8	3	13
1984	9	12	1	13
1985	14	33	1	15
1986	17	37	2	13
1987[a]	15	37	1	11

Abbreviations: AV, aortic valve; MV, mitral valve.
[a] Data for January 1 through June 30, 1987.
Data from Ballard DJ, Khandheria BK, Tajik AJ, et al. A population-based study of echocardiography: secular trends in utilization and diagnostic profile of an evolving technology 1975–1987. Int J Technology Assessment Health Care 1989;5(2):249–61.

are the principal and secondary discharge diagnoses and the principal and secondary in-patient procedures, coded according to the International Classification of Disease, Version 9 (ICD-9) classification system. The authors analyzed all records that contained principal or secondary ICD-9 codes reflecting diseases of the mitral or aortic valve, diseases of the mitral and aortic valve, or diseases of other endocardial structures (including the tricuspid and pulmonic valves). For purposes of comparison, the authors also examined trends in the total number of hospitalizations in New York State during the same period [82].

In total, more than 1 million cases of VHD were identified among New York State in-patients. Approximately 40% of these patients were hospitalized during the last 5 years of data collection. Average age of the population was 65 years at hospital discharge or death. Age increased sharply between 1983 and 2000. Most patients had clinical diagnoses of mitral or aortic valve disease (mostly nonrheumatic), with mitral disease predominating. Relatively few patients had combined disease of these two valves; even fewer had tricuspid or pulmonic valve disease. Mitral valve disease was found principally among relatively younger white women, whereas prevalence of aortic valve disease was greatest among white men. Although hospitalizations in New York State decreased progressively and linearly during the 18-year interval, the incidence of hospitalizations of patients diagnosed with VHD increased approximately threefold during the same period (Fig. 5). The rates of increase were

approximately linear for all forms of VHD and were documented among all demographic subgroups (men and women, whites and nonwhites, older and younger patients). The rate of increase for mitral valve disease (MR or MS), however, was 1.5-fold greater than the rate observed for aortic valve disease (AR or AS) and was appreciably greater than rates observed for tricuspid or pulmonic valve diseases [82].

More than 80,000 therapeutic valve procedures (predominantly valve replacement; less commonly open chest valvotomy, other open chest repair, and percutaneous balloon valvuloplasty) were performed in New York State between 1983 and 2000 among in-patients. The numbers of these procedures increased almost linearly during this period (Fig. 6). Valve surgery rates increased more rapidly among patients 65 years or older versus younger patients and among men versus women. No disparities were found in the rate of surgery among white versus nonwhite patients [82].

Approximately 63,000 in-patients who had VHDs died in New York State hospitals during the 18-year study interval. Deaths more than doubled between 1983 and 2000. When the number of deaths was adjusted for the number of patients hospitalized with VHDs, however, mortality rates remained constant at approximately 5.4% per year, despite generally recognized advances in health care technology and delivery [82]. Data were not sufficient to compare VHD hospital death rates with rates due to other cardiovascular diseases or to confidently identify independent predisposing factors. Nonetheless, it

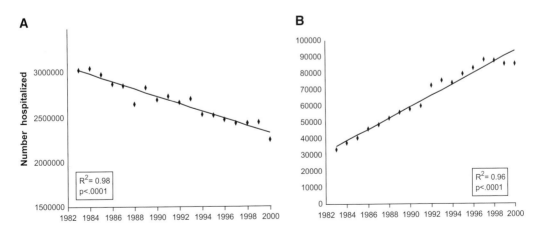

Fig. 5. Temporal changes in number of hospitalizations in New York State between 1983 and 2000. (*A*) Total number of hospitalizations (all causes) versus (*B*) hospitalizations including a VHD diagnosis (mitral, aortic, tricuspid, or pulmonic valve diseases). (*From* Supino PG, Borer JS, Yin A, et al. The epidemiology of valvular heart diseases: the problem is growing. Adv Cardiol 2004;41:11; with permission. Copyright 2004, S. Karger AG, Basel.)

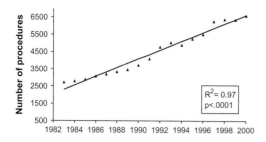

Fig. 6. Temporal change in number of therapeutic valve procedures performed between 1983 and 2000 in New York State. Procedures include open chest valvotomy or other valve repair, valve replacement, and percutaneous balloon valvuloplasty. (*From* Supino PG, Borer JS, Yin A, et al. The epidemiology of valvular heart diseases: the problem is growing. Adv Cardiol 2004;41:12; with permission. Copyright 2004, S. Karger AG, Basel.)

is reasonable to speculate that these relatively high mortality statistics may result from increasing numbers of elderly patients who have more advanced VHD and other comorbidities who are being treated in our hospitals.

The increase in VHD hospitalization and surgical procedures revealed by the SPARCS data was confirmed by Otto [84] in her recent analysis of hospital discharges and heart valve surgeries throughout the United States between 1985 and 1999. These data showed approximately linear increases in the number of discharge diagnoses of nonrheumatic mitral and aortic valve disease during this period, with nonrheumatic mitral disease predominating. Significant increases also were noted in the number of diagnoses of rheumatic MR but not in MS or endocarditis (Fig. 7), resulting in approximately 1 million total VHD diagnoses in 1999. Again, consistent with the SPARCS data, marked increases were noted in the number of surgical valve procedures performed in the United States (approximately 80,000 in 1999, excluding percutaneous valvuloplasty; Fig. 8) [84]. Temporal trends in mortality and in demographically defined subgroups were not evaluated.

Summary

Cross-sectional data indicate that VHDs are present in a relatively large proportion of our population. In many cases, the VHDs now being recognized are of only mild severity. Nonetheless, a substantial number of individuals in the United States currently manifest VHD (predominantly

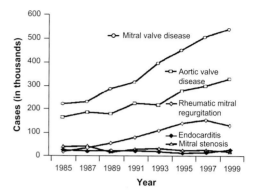

Fig. 7. Number of all discharge diagnoses of VHD in the United States between 1985 and 1999 based on the National Center for Health Statistics ICD-9-M discharge code data, available at www.cdc.gov/nchs. (*From* Otto CM. Valvular heart disease. 2nd edition. Philadelphia: WB Saunders; 2004. p. 2; with permission. Copyright 2004, Elsevier, Inc.)

nonrheumatic) that is moderate or severe, potentially warranting intervention. Although it is unclear whether the observed temporal patterns are due to better detection, increased prevalence, severity of illness, or a combination of these factors, longitudinal studies show that echocardiographic and clinical diagnoses of VHDs among inpatients have increased markedly in the United States since the early 1980s, as have mechanical

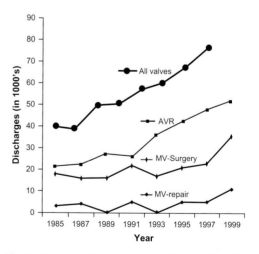

Fig. 8. Number of heart valve procedures performed in the United States between 1985 and 1999 based on the National Center for Health Statistics ICD-9-CM procedure codes. AVR, aortic valve replacement. (*From* Otto CM. Valvular heart disease. 2nd edition. Philadelphia: WB Saunders; 2004. p. 2; with permission. Copyright 2004, Elsevier, Inc.)

interventions designed to correct these disorders. The patterns reported herein are sufficiently pronounced, consistent, and sustained so that the increase in VHD-associated hospitalizations, aggressive treatments, and severe sequelae are likely to continue as the population ages and expands. Increasingly, research and health care resources should be targeted toward meeting this important public health challenge.

References

[1] Wilson PWF. An epidemiologic perspective of systemic hypertension, ischemic heart disease, and heart failure. Am J Cardiol 1997;80(9B):3J–8J.

[2] Mangion JR, Tighe DA. Aortic valvular disease in adults. Postgrad Med 1995;98(1):127–40.

[3] Grigioni F, Enriquez-Sarano M, Ling LH, et al. Sudden death in mitral regurgitation due to flail leaflet. J Am Coll Cardiol 1999;34(7):2078–85.

[4] Thom T, Haase N, Rosamond W, et al. Heart disease and stroke statistics—2006 update: a report from the American Heart Association Statistical Committee and Stroke Statistics Subcommittee. Circulation 2006;113(6):85–121.

[5] Reid CL, Gardin JM, Yunis C, et al. Prevalence and clinical correlates of aortic and mitral regurgitation in a young population. The Cardia Study. Circulation 1994;90(4):I-282.

[6] Singh JP, Evans JC, Levy D, et al. Prevalence and clinical determinants of mitral, tricuspid and aortic regurgitation (the Framingham Heart Study). Am J Cardiol 1999;83(6):897–902.

[7] Jones EC, Devereux RB, Roman MJ, et al. Prevalence and correlates of mitral regurgitation in a population-based sample (the Strong Heart Study). Am J Cardiol 2001;87(3):298–304.

[8] Follman DF. Aortic regurgitation: identifying and treating acute and chronic disease. Postgrad Med 1993;93(6):83–90.

[9] Hochreiter C, Niles N, Devereux RB, et al. Mitral regurgitation: relationship of noninvasive descriptors of right and left ventricular performance to clinical and hemodynamic findings and to prognosis in medically and surgically treated patients. Circulation 1986;73(5):900–12.

[10] Borer JS, Hochreiter C, Herrold EM, et al. Prediction of indications for valve replacement among asymptomatic or minimally symptomatic patients with chronic aortic regurgitation and normal left ventricular performance. Circulation 1998;97(6): 525–34.

[11] Glancy DL. Mitral stenosis: 1. Anatomical, physiological, and clinical considerations. J La State Med Soc 2003;155(2):91–5.

[12] Carabello BA. Is it ever too late to operate on the patient with valvular heart disease? J Am Coll Cardiol 2004;44(2):376–83.

[13] Sabet HY, Edwards WD, Tazelaar HD, et al. Congenitally bicuspid aortic valves: a surgical pathology study of 542 cases (1991 through 1996) and a literature review of 2,715 additional cases. Mayo Clin Proc 1999;74(1):14–26.

[14] Ross J Jr, Braunwald E. Aortic stenosis. Circulation 1968;38(Suppl 1):61–7.

[15] Park MH. Timely intervention in asymptomatic aortic stenosis. Emerging clinical parameters may help predict outcomes. Postgrad Med 2001;110(2): 28–39.

[16] Aronow WS, Ahn C, Kronzon I. Prevalence of echocardiographic findings in 554 men and in 1,243 women aged > 60 years in a long-term health facility. Am J Cardiol 1997;79(3):379–80.

[17] Aronow WS. Prevalence of heart disease in older women in a nursing home. J Womens Health 1998; 7(9):1105–12.

[18] Lindroos M, Kupari M, Heikkila J, et al. Prevalence of aortic valve abnormalities in the elderly: an echocardiographic study of a random population sample. J Am Coll Cardiol 1993;21(5):1220–5.

[19] Stewart BF, Siscovick D, Lind BK, et al. Clinical factors associated with calcific aortic valve disease. J Am Coll Cardiol 1997;29(3):630–4.

[20] Carabello BA, Crawford FA Jr. Valvular heart disease. N Engl J Med 1997;337(1):32–41.

[21] Alpert JS. Chronic aortic regurgitation. In: Dalen JE, Alpert JS, editors. Valvular heart disease. 2nd edition. Boston: Little, Brown and Co.; 1987. p. 283–318.

[22] Siemienczuk D, Greenberg B, Morris C, et al. Chronic aortic insufficiency: factors associated with progression to aortic valve replacement. Ann Intern Med 1989;110(8):587–92.

[23] Bonow RO, Lakatos E, Maron BJ, et al. Serial long-term assessment of the natural history of asymptomatic patients with chronic aortic regurgitation and normal left ventricular systolic function. Circulation 1991;84(4):1625–35.

[24] Morganroth J, Perloff JK, Zeldis SM, et al. Acute severe aortic regurgitation: pathophysiology, clinical recognition, and management. Ann Intern Med 1977;87(2):223–32.

[25] Kostucki W, Vandenbossche J-L, Friart A, et al. Pulsed Doppler regurgitant flow patterns of normal valves. Am J Cardiol 1986;58(3):309–13.

[26] Akasaka T, Yoshikawa J, Yoshida K, et al. Age-related valvular regurgitation: a study by pulsed Doppler echocardiography. Circulation 1987;76(2):262–5.

[27] Yoshida K, Yoshikawa J, Shakudo M, et al. Color Doppler evaluation of valvular regurgitation in normal subjects. Circulation 1988;78(4):840–7.

[28] Berger M, Hecht SR, Van Tosh A, et al. Pulsed and continuous wave Doppler echocardiographic assessment of valvular regurgitation in normal subjects. J Am Coll Cardiol 1989;13(7):1540–5.

[29] Choong CY, Abascal VM, Weyman J, et al. Prevalence of valvular regurgitation by Doppler echocardiography in patients with structurally normal

hearts by two-dimensional echocardiography. Am Heart J 1989;117(3):636–42.

[30] Klein AL, Burstow DJ, Tajik AJ, et al. Age-related prevalence of valvular regurgitation in normal subjects: a comprehensive color flow examination of 118 volunteers. J Am Soc Echo 1990;2(1):54–63.

[31] Brand A, Dollberg S, Keren A. The prevalence of valvular regurgitation in children with structurally normal hearts: a color Doppler echocardiographic study. Am Heart J 1992;123(1):177–80.

[32] Lavie CJ, Hebert K, Cassidy M. Prevalence and severity of Doppler-detected valvular regurgitation and estimation of right-sided cardiac pressures in patients with normal two-dimensional echocardiograms. Chest 1993;103(1):226–31.

[33] Lebowitz NE, Bella JN, Roman MJ, et al. Prevalence and correlates of aortic regurgitation in American Indians: the Strong Heart Study. J Am Coll Cardiol 2000;36(2):461–7.

[34] Olson LJ, Subramanian R, Ackermann DM, et al. Surgical pathology of the mitral valve: a study of 712 cases spanning 21 years. Mayo Clin Proc 1987; 62(1):22–34.

[35] Adabag AS, Dykoski R, Ward H, et al. Critical stenosis of aortic and mitral valves after mediastinal irradiation. Catheter Cardiovasc Interv 2004;63(2): 247–50.

[36] Braunwald E. Valvular heart disease. In: Braunwald E, editor. Heart disease: a textbook of cardiovascular medicine. 5th edition. Philadelphia: WB Saunders; 1997. p. 1007–61.

[37] Feldman T. Rheumatic mitral stenosis. On the rise again. Postgrad Med 1993;93(6):93–104.

[38] Carroll JD, Feldman T. Percutaneous mitral balloon valvotomy and the new demographics of mitral stenosis. JAMA 1993;270(14):1731–6.

[39] Carabello BA. Modern management of mitral stenosis. Circulation 2005;112(3):432–7.

[40] Homer C, Shulman ST. Clinical aspects of acute rheumatic fever. J Rheumatol 1991;18(Suppl 29): 2–13.

[41] Ayoub EM. Resurgence of rheumatic fever in the United States. The changing picture of a preventable illness. Postgrad Med 1992;92(3):133–42.

[42] Griffiths SP, Gersony WM. Acute rheumatic fever in New York City (1969 to 1988): a comparative study of two decades. J Pediatr 1990;116(6):882–7.

[43] Westlake RM, Graham TP, Edwards KM. An outbreak of acute rheumatic fever in Tennessee. Pediatr Infect Dis J 1990;9(1):97–100.

[44] Wald ER, Dashefsky B, Feidt C, et al. Acute rheumatic fever in western Pennsylvania and the Tri-State area. Pediatrics 1987;80(3):371–4.

[45] Congeni B, Rizzo C, Congeni J, et al. Outbreak of acute rheumatic fever in northeast Ohio. J Pediatr 1987;111(2):176–9.

[46] Centers for Disease Control. Acute rheumatic fever at a navy training center-San Diego, California. MMWR Morb Mortal Wkly Rep 1988;37(7):101–4.

[47] Horstkotte D, Niehues R, Strauer BE. Pathomorphological aspects, aetiology and natural history of acquired mitral valve stenosis. Eur Heart J 1991; 12(Suppl B):55–60.

[48] Stollerman GH. Rheumatic fever and other rheumatic disease of the heart. In: Braunwald E, editor. Heart disease: a textbook of cardiovascular medicine. 4th edition. Philadelphia: Saunders Co; 1992. p. 1721–31.

[49] Rosen SE, Borer JS, Hochreiter C, et al. Natural history of the asymptomatic/minimally symptomatic patient with severe mitral regurgitation secondary to mitral valve prolapse and normal right and left ventricular performance. Am J Cardiol 1994;74(4): 374–80.

[50] Enriquez-Sarano M, Avierinos JF, Messika-Zeitoun D, et al. Quantitative determinants of the outcome of asymptomatic mitral regurgitation. N Engl J Med 2005;352(9):875–83.

[51] Scott RL. Native mitral valve regurgitation. Postgrad Med 2001;110(2):57–63.

[52] Flack JM, Kvasnicka JH, Gardin JM, et al, for the CARDIA investigators. Anthropometric and physiological correlates of mitral valve prolapse in a biethnic cohort of young adults: the CARDIA Study. Am Heart J 1999;138(3):486–92.

[53] Ockene IS. Tricuspid valve disease. In: Dalen JE, Alpert JS, editors. Valvular heart disease. 2nd edition. Boston: Little, Brown and Co.; 1987. p. 353–402.

[54] Poveda JJ, Bernal JM, Matorras P, et al. Tricuspid valve replacement in rheumatic disease: preoperative predictors of hospital mortality. J Heart Valve Dis 1996;5(1):26–30.

[55] Kitchin A, Turner R. Diagnosis and treatment of tricuspid stenosis. Br Heart J 1964;26:354–79.

[56] Bailey CP, Bolton HE. Criteria for and results of surgery for mitral stenosis. Part II. Results of mitral commissurotomy. N Y St J Med 1956;56(5): 825–39.

[57] Goswami KC, Rao MB, Dev V, et al. Juvenile tricuspid stenosis and rheumatic tricuspid valve disease: an echocardiographic study. Int J Cardiol 1999;72(1): 83–6.

[58] Chockalingam A, Gnanavelu G, Elangovan S, et al. Clinical spectrum of chronic rheumatic heart disease in India. J Heart Valve Dis 2003;12(5):577–81.

[59] Salazar E, Levine HD. Rheumatic tricuspid regurgitation: the clinical spectrum. Am J Med 1962;33: 111–29.

[60] Kim HK, Kim YJ, Park JS, et al. Determinants of the severity of functional tricuspid regurgitation. Am J Cardiol 2006;98(2):236–42.

[61] Connolly HM, Crary JL, McGoon MD, et al. Valvular heart disease associated with fenfluramine-phentermine. N Engl J Med 1997;337(9):581–8.

[62] Raman SV, Sparks EA, Boudoulas H, et al. Tricuspid valve disease: tricuspid valve complex perspective. Curr Probl Cardiol 2002;27(3):103–42.

[63] Nath J, Foster E, Heidenreich PA. Impact of triscuspid regurgitation on long-term survival. J Am Coll Cardiol 2004;43(3):405–9.

[64] Yankah AC, Musci M, Weng Y, et al. Tricuspid valve dysfunction and surgery after orthotopic cardiac transplantation. Eur J Cardiothorac Surg 2000;17(4):343–8.

[65] Akasaka T, Lythall DA, Kushwaha SS, et al. Valvular regurgitation in heart-lung transplant recipients: a Doppler color flow study. J Am Coll Cardiol 1990; 15(3):576–81.

[66] Nguyen V, Cantarovich M, Cecere R, et al. Tricuspid regurgitation after cardiac transplantation: how many biopsies are too many? J Heart Lung Transplant 2005;24(Suppl 7):S227–31.

[67] Valdes-Cruz LM, Cayre RO. Anomalies of the right ventricular outflow tract and pulmonary arteries. In: Valdes-Cruz LM, Cayre RO, editors. Echocardiographic diagnosis of congenital heart disease. An embryologic and anatomic approach. Philadelphia: Lippincott-Raven; 1999. p. 325–48.

[68] Rao PS. Pulmonic valve disease. In: Alpert JS, Dalen J, Rahimtoola S, editors. Valvular heart disease. 3rd edition. Philadelphia: Lippincott, Williams & Wilkins; 2000. p. 339–76.

[69] Johnson LW, Grossman W, Dalen JE, et al. Pulmonic stenosis in the adult. N Engl J Med 1972; 287(23):1159–63.

[70] Ferencz C, Rubin JD, McCarter RJ, et al. Congenital heart disease: prevalence at live birth. The Baltimore-Washington Infant Study. Am J Epidemiol 1985;121(1):31–6.

[71] Samanek M, Slavik Z, Zborilova B, et al. Prevalence, treatment, and outcome of heart disease in live-born children: a prospective analysis of 91,823 live-born children. Pediatr Cardiol 1989;10(4):205–11.

[72] Grech V. History, diagnosis, surgery and epidemiology of pulmonary stenosis in Malta. Cardiol Young 1998;8(3):337–43.

[73] Geva T, Sandweiss BM, Gauvreau K, et al. Factors associated with impaired clinical status in long-term survivors of tetralogy of Fallot repair evaluated by magnetic resonance imaging. J Am Coll Cardiol 2004;43(6):1068–74.

[74] Bouzas B, Kilner PJ, Gatzoulis MA. Pulmonary regurgitation: not a benign lesion. Eur Heart J 2005; 26(5):433–9.

[75] Akram M, Khan IA. Isolated pulmonic valve endocarditis caused by group B streptococcus (*Streptococcus agalactiae*). A case report and literature review. Angiology 2001;52(3):211–5.

[76] Liuzzo JP, Shin YT, Lucariello R, et al. Triple valve repair for rheumatic heart disease. J Card Surg 2005; 20(4):358–63.

[77] Connolly HM, Schaff HV, Mullany CJ, et al. Carcinoid heart disease: impact of pulmonary valve replacement in right ventricular function and remodeling. Circulation 2002;106(Suppl 12):I51–6.

[78] Nathan D, Kraus J, Deutsch V, et al. Dilation of the aorta and pulmonary artery with aortic and pulmonary insufficiency in the presence of a ventricular septal defect and infundibular pulmonic stenosis. Report of a case of forme fruste of the Marfan syndrome. Dis Chest 1966;50(2):199–205.

[79] de Ruijter FT, Weenink I, Hitchcock J, et al. Right ventricular dysfunction and pulmonary valve replacement after correction of tetralogy of Fallot. Ann Thorac Surg 2002;73(6):1794–800 [discussion: 1800].

[80] Supino PG, Borer JS, Yin A. The epidemiology of valvular heart disease: an emerging public health problem. Adv Cardiol 2002;39:1–6.

[81] Ballard DJ, Khandheria BK, Tajik AJ, et al. Population-based study of echocardiography: time trends in utilization and diagnostic profile of an evolving technology 1975–1987. Int J Technol Assess Health Care 1989;5(2):249–61.

[82] Supino PG, Borer JS, Yin A, et al. The epidemiology of valvular heart diseases: the problem is growing. Adv Cardiol 2004;41:9–15.

[83] Quan JM. SPARCS: the New York State Health Care Data System. J Clin Comput 1980;8(6):255–63.

[84] Otto CM. Valvular heart disease. 2nd edition. Philadelphia: WB Saunders; 2004.

ELSEVIER
SAUNDERS

Heart Failure Clin 2 (2006) 395–413

HEART
FAILURE
CLINICS

Role of Statins in Aortic Valve Disease

Nalini M. Rajamannan, MD, FACC, FAHA[a,b,*]

[a]Northwestern University Feinberg School of Medicine, Chicago, IL, USA
[b]Bluhm Cardiovascular Institute, Northwestern Memorial Hospital, Chicago, IL, USA

Calcific aortic stenosis is the most common indication for surgical valve replacement in the United States [1]. Currently, in 2006, surgical valve replacement is the only treatment for this disease process [2]. For years, this disease has been described as a passive process that develops secondary to serum calcium attaching to the valve leaflet surface to cause nodule formation. Therefore, surgical replacement of the valve is the obvious approach toward relieving outflow obstruction in these patients. Severe aortic stenosis causes progressive left ventricular hypertrophy, left ventricular diastolic and systolic dysfunction, congestive heart failure, angina, arrhythmias, and syncope. Recent studies demonstrate an association between atherosclerosis and its risk factors and aortic valve disease. Although a unifying hypothesis for the role of atherosclerotic risk factors in the mechanism of vascular and aortic valve disease is emerging, progress in studying the cell biology of this disease has been limited in the past by the paucity of experimental models available.

In 2006, a number of epidemiologic and experimental studies provided evidence that this disease process is not a passive phenomenon. Moreover, the histologic and experimental models indicate that there is an active cellular biology that develops within the valve leaflet and causes a regulated bone formation to occur. A similar paradigm shift occurred in the last part of the twentieth century in the field of vascular disease. Vascular atherosclerosis, once thought to be a "degenerative process," is now an active biologic process that

can be targeted with medical therapy. A similar phenomenon has occurred with aortic valve disease and with the growing number of clinical and experimental studies over the past decade. The growing evidence for the etiology of degenerative calcific aortic valve disease points toward a "response to injury" mechanism similar to what has been described for vascular atherosclerosis.

If the atherosclerotic hypothesis is present in the development of aortic stenosis, then treatments used in slowing the progression of vascular atherosclerosis may be effective in patients who have aortic valve disease. Current management of calcific aortic valve disease focuses on defining patients who have valvular disease and the development of symptoms to determine the timing of surgical valve replacement. This article reviews the pathogenesis and the potential for medical therapy in the management of patients who have calcific aortic stenosis. It provides an overview of the emerging experimental and clinical studies important in the understanding of the cellular mechanisms of this disease process. It also addresses the growing number of retrospective and prospective clinical studies evaluating the use of statins as a potential for cholesterol lowering treatment to prevent progression of aortic valve calcification.

The role for lipids and signaling pathways in atherosclerosis in aortic valve disease

Vascular atherosclerosis has been described in the literature for hundreds of years [3]. In 2006, the complexity of atherosclerosis and the different signaling pathways involved in the development of this pathology were under intense investigation, including (1) lipid signaling pathways in the vascular wall [4–6], (2) evaluation of an immune

* Department of Cardiology, Northwestern University Feinberg School of Medicine, 303 E. Chicago Avenue, Tarry 12-717, Chicago, IL 60611.
E-mail address: n-rajamannan@northwestern.edu

1551-7136/06/$ - see front matter © 2007 Elsevier Inc. All rights reserved.
doi:10.1016/j.hfc.2006.09.011

hypothesis for the mechanism of vascular inflammation [7,8], (3) identification of cytokines and chemokines [9], (4) determination of the effects of macrophages and T-cell activation in the vessel wall [5,10], and (5) effects of lipoprotein and insulin metabolism and their interactions with the vessel wall—all resulting in a multifactorial approach toward studying the mechanisms of vascular atherosclerosis [11].

Emerging epidemiologic studies are revealing convincing clinical evidence toward an atherosclerotic hypothesis for the cellular mechanism of this valvular lesion. Risk factors for calcific aortic valve disease have recently been described, including male sex, hypertension, elevated levels of low-density lipoprotein (LDL), and smoking [12–22]. These risk factors are similar to those that promote the development of vascular atherosclerosis [23–25]. Table 1 demonstrates the retrospective studies implicating vascular risk factors for atherosclerosis. Surgical pathologic studies have demonstrated the presence of LDL [26,27] and atherosclerosis in calcified human aortic valves, demonstrating similarities between the genesis of valvular and vascular disease and suggesting a common cellular mechanism of atherosclerosis in these tissues [27]. Fig. 1 demonstrates the immunohistochemistry by O'Brien and colleagues [27] showing the presence of apolipoproteins present in cardiac valves from patients who have early valvular heart disease. This study, confirmed by Olsson and colleagues [26], proved that lipoproteins are present in the development of calcific aortic valve disease. Recent evidence demonstrating the presence of (hs)C-reactive protein in valve

specimens also indicates that valvular stenosis is an inflammatory state [28–30]. The role of hypercholesterolemia in vascular and valvular atherosclerosis induces an inflammatory environment that can lead to an activation of inflammatory signaling pathways. Studies have tested one of the growing numbers of signaling pathways: the effect of transforming growth factor β in calcified aortic valves [31,32]. Many of these studies show that transforming growth factor β is important in the activation of the valve myofibroblasts cells to undergo the differentiation process to calcification.

Clinically, the correlation of hypercholesterolemia and valvular disease has been well described in the patients who have familial hypercholesterolemia (FH). This patient population develops accelerated atherosclerosis within the entire vasculature and cardiac valves. Autopsy studies of these patients demonstrate a severe form of aortic stenosis associated with supravalvar narrowing [33]. In this specific condition, extremely high LDL cholesterol concentrations are seen without the other traditional risk factors for coronary artery disease. Recently, the proof of principle for the atherosclerotic process was demonstrated in a case report from a patient born in 1942 [34]. In this study, Rajamannan and colleagues [34] reported a patient with the diagnosis of FH IIb and prominent skin xanthomas at the time of birth. The patient died of cardiac complications at age 7 years and had an elevated cholesterol level of greater than 900 mg/dL. Rajamannan and colleagues [34] examined the cardiac pathology that demonstrated coronary atherosclerosis and aortic valve atherosclerosis.

Table 1
Risk factors associated with aortic stenosis

Study	Study design	N	Mean age	Positive risk factors
Deutscher et al, 1984 [12]	Case control	54	NA	Lipids, diabetes
Hoagland et al, 1985 [73]	Case control	105	66	None
Aronow et al, 1987 [13]	Hospital survey	571	82	HTN, lipids, DM, low HDL
Mohler et al, 1991 [14]	Retrospective	39 BAV	62	Sex, low TRG, smoking, race
Lindroos et al, 1994 [15]	Prospective	501	75	HTN, low BMI
Boon et al, 1997 [16]	Retrospective	515	67	Age, HTN, lipids
Stewart et al, 1997 [17]	Prospective	5201	73	Sex, age, HTN, Lp(a), LDL chol
Wilmshurst et al, 1997 [18]	Prospective	20 D; 6 BAV	66	Lipids
Chan et al, 2001 [19]	Prospective	48 BAV	56	Lipids
Aronow et al, 2001 [20]	Retrospective	180	82	Sex, smoking, HTN, DM, lipids
Chui et al, 2001 [21]	Retrospective	43 D	66	Lipids
Peltier et al, 2003 [22]	Prospective	220	68	HTN, smoking, high BMI, lipids

Abbreviations: BAV, bicuspid; BMI, body mass index; D, tricuspid; DM, diabetes mellitus; HTN, hypertension; LDL chol, LDL cholesterol; Lp (a), lipoprotein (a); NA, not applicable; TRG, triglycerides.

Data from Chan KL. Is aortic stenosis a preventable disease? J Am Coll Cardiol 2003;42(4):596.

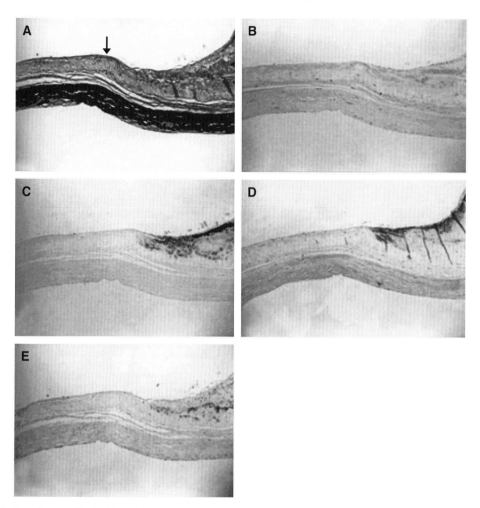

Fig. 1. Apoplipoproteins B, (a), and E accumulate in the morphologically early lesion of "degenerative" valvular aortic stenosis (*A–E*). (*From* O'Brien KD, Reichenbach DD, Marcovina SM, et al. Apolipoproteins B, (a), and E accumulate in the morphologically early lesion of 'degenerative' valvular aortic stenosis. Arterioscler Thromb Vasc Biol 1996;16(4):524; with permission.)

Fig. 2 demonstrates the development of atherosclerosis along the aortic surface of the aortic valve and in the lumen of the left circumflex [34]. This study and previous studies of this patient population [33–37] have provided the descriptive proof of atherosclerosis involving the vascular and valvular structures, providing further proof that valvular heart disease involves a similar pathophysiology of vascular atherosclerosis.

Experimental models of valvular atherosclerosis

There are emerging experimental in vivo models evaluating the effects of experimental hypercholesterolemia on atherosclerosis in the aortic valves [38–41]. The rabbit model of feeding a high-cholesterol diet has been used for years in the field of vascular atherosclerosis. The author's laboratory has developed the rabbit model of experimental hypercholesterolemia inducing valvular heart disease. Early studies demonstrate that the vascular lesion in the rabbit aorta from experimental hypercholesterolemia has a similar atherosclerotic lesion of that of the aortic valve [39]. After 8 weeks of 1.0% cholesterol diet, the aortic valves and aortas from these rabbits develop a similar atherosclerosis lesion. Fig. 3 shows the comparison of the vascular aorta to the aortic valve from this rabbit model.

Left Circumflex Artery **Aortic Valve**

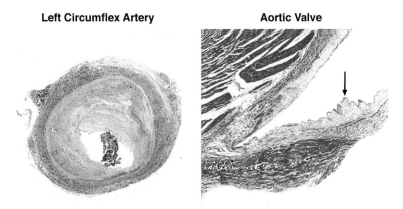

Fig. 2. Hypercholesterolemic aortic valve disease. Development of atherosclerosis in the lumen of the left circumflex (*left*) and along the aortic surface of the aortic valve (*right*). The arrow points to the atherosclerotic lesion along the aortic valve surface. (*From* Rajamannan NM, Edwards WD, Spelsberg TC. Hypercholesterolemic aortic-valve disease. N Engl J Med 2003;349(7):717; with permission. Copyright © 2003, Massachusetts Medical Society.)

Fig. 3A is the normal aorta and the aortic valve, demonstrating a clear aortic valve leaflet and normal appearing aorta. Fig. 3B is the hypercholesterolemic aorta and aortic valve, demonstrating marked exudative lesions along the aortic surface of the valve and extending along the aorta. Fig. 3C is the longitudinal cross-section of the normal-diet aortic valve attached to the aorta with no evidence of atherosclerosis. Fig. 3D demonstrates the fatty streak lesion along the aortic surface and indicates the atherosclerotic lesion along the valve leaflet. Fig. 3E demonstrates a cross-sectional view of the proximal thoracic aorta, which is normal in the control diet. Fig. 3F demonstrates the atherosclerotic lesion in the vascular aorta and indicates the fatty streak atheromatous lesion in the lumen. Further analysis of this early aortic valve lesion identified apoptosis and cellular proliferation present in the atherosclerotic valve lesion [39]. Drolet and colleagues [38] also tested an experimental diet including vitamin D and hypercholesterolemia in mice. They found that the diet induces a hemodynamic early stenotic lesion within the aortic valve leaflets, which was confirmed by echocardiography. Fig. 4 demonstrates the continuous wave Doppler waveform across the stenotic aortic valve of the rabbits treated with control versus vitamin D plus cholesterol. Atherosclerosis and foam cell formation are the hallmarks of vascular atherosclerosis. The rabbit and genetic mouse models are serving as the future foundation for the evaluation of the cellular pathways and mechanisms of the development of valvular heart disease.

Aortic valve calcification as the final common pathway to surgical valve replacement

Understanding calcification is the key to the success of understanding aortic valve stenosis. Calcification is a common feature of vascular atherosclerotic plaques and stenotic aortic valves. The presence of calcification may lead to clinical vascular complications, including myocardial infarction, impaired vascular tone, and coronary insufficiency caused by loss of aortic recoil [42]. Calcification in the aortic valve is the final common pathway that leads to aortic valve stenosis. This finding was confirmed in an echocardiographic study demonstrating that patients who have severe aortic stenosis and severe calcification have a worse prognosis than patients who have mild calcification and severe aortic stenosis [43]. The data further corroborate the evidence that calcification is the clinically defining feature of prognostic implications for this patient population.

Recent intriguing observations suggest that rapid advancement in our understanding of the basic mechanisms involved in the initiation and progression of vascular and valvular calcification is now possible. Historically, cardiovascular calcification was considered a degenerative process leading to passive accumulation of calcium phosphate. New findings strongly suggest that ectopic mineralization is part of an active ongoing process rather than the result of passive degeneration. The concept of regulated vascular calcification suggests the presence of cellular and molecular

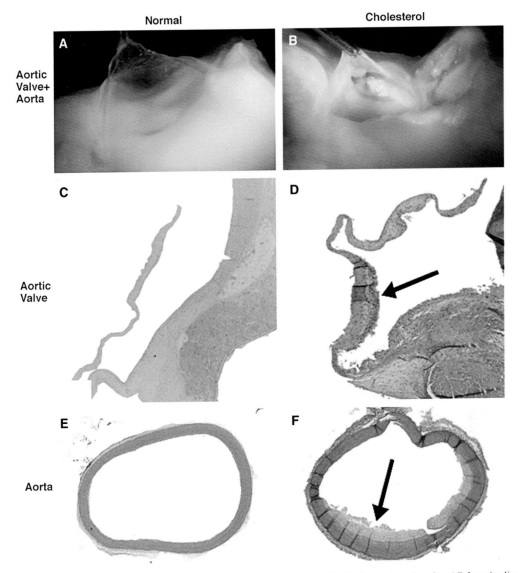

Fig. 3. Atherosclerotic aortic valve versus aorta. (*A*) Control aortic valve. (*B*) Cholesterol aortic valve. (*C*) Longitudinal cross-section of control aorta and aortic valve. (*D*) Longitudinal cross-section of cholesterol aorta and aortic valve. Arrow points to the atherosclerotic lesion along the aortic valve surface. (*E*) Control proximal aorta. (*F*) Cholesterol proximal aorta. Arrow points to the atherosclerotic lesion along the proximal aorta.

determinants of ectopic calcification, natural inhibitors of ectopic calcification, and regulators of bone resorption.

Most research has evolved around descriptive histologic and protein expression studies delineating the development of calcification in the aortic valve. Studies have shown that cardiovascular calcification is composed of hydroxyapatite deposited on a bonelike matrix of collagen, osteopontin, and other minor bone matrix proteins

[44–46]. In addition, osteopontin expression has been demonstrated in the mineralization zones of heavily calcified aortic valves obtained at autopsy and surgery [43,46]. Mohler and colleagues [44,45] were the first to confirm histologically the presence of osteoblast bone formation in calcified aortic valves removed from surgical valve replacement. Fig. 5 demonstrates inflammation and histologic characteristics of bone formation in the calcified cardiac valves from this study.

Control

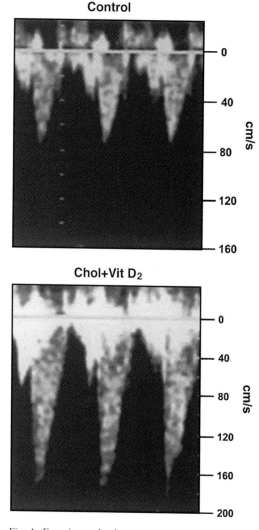

Chol+Vit D₂

Fig. 4. Experimental valve stenosis in rabbits. Continuous wave Doppler waveform across the stenotic aortic valve of rabbits treated with control (*top*) versus vitamin D plus cholesterol (*bottom*). (*From* Drolet MC, Arsenault M, Couet J. Experimental aortic valve stenosis in rabbits. J Am Coll Cardiol 2003;41(7):1215; with permission. Copyright © 2003, American College of Cardiology Foundation.)

The author's laboratory has demonstrated by reverse transcriptase polymerase chain reaction analysis, by histomorphometry, and by microCT that an osteoblast-like cellular phenotype is present in calcified aortic valves removed at the time of surgical valve replacement [47].

In this study by Rajamannan and colleagues [47], human calcified valves demonstrated evidence of mineralization in the valve leaflets by

contact microradiography (Fig. 6A). This finding of calcification was supported with histologic staining to confirm the presence of mineralization in calcified valve tissues. The microradiograph in Fig. 6B depicts two areas of calcification in the valve leaflet. Goldner's Modified Masson trichrome stain demonstrates an increase in green stain, indicating an increase with hydroxyapatite synthesis around the areas of heavy calcification (Fig. 6B and C). The von Kossa technique stains calcium crystals black, following a similar pattern as in Goldner's Modified Masson trichrome green stain (see Fig. 6D and E).

Rajamannan and colleagues [47] also tested mRNA from calcified versus normal aortic valves to determine osteoblast markers in calcified aortic valves, including osteopontin, bone sialoprotein, osteocalcin, alkaline phosphatase, and the osteoblast-specific transcription factor Cbfa1. Fig. 7 demonstrates that all markers except for alkaline phosphatase were increased in the calcified aortic valves compared with the noncalcified controls.

These ex vivo and in vivo models have provided a basic novel understanding of the development of calcification in the aortic valve and may represent parallel signaling pathways that are present in aortic valve myofibroblast cells and osteoblast cells. Furthermore, these studies demonstrate that the aortic valve may have a bone biology instead of a passive degenerative process.

LDL receptor–related protein 5 signaling pathway in the development of valvular heart disease

Studies have recently shown that different mutations in LDL receptor–related protein 5 (Lrp5) develop a high bone mass phenotype and an osteoporosis phenotype, implicating this coreceptor and the canonical Wnt signaling pathway in bone formation and bone mass regulation [48,49]. The author's laboratory and others have recently demonstrated in experimental animal models that bone matrix protein expression in the aortic valve and vasculature are regulated by the Lrp5 pathway in the presence of elevated hypercholesterolemia [50,51]. The Lrp5, a coreceptor of the LDL receptor family, has been discovered as an important receptor in the activation of skeletal bone formation by way of binding to the secreted glycoprotein Wnt (a growth factor) and activating β-catenin to induce bone formation. Therefore, the author and colleagues hypothesized

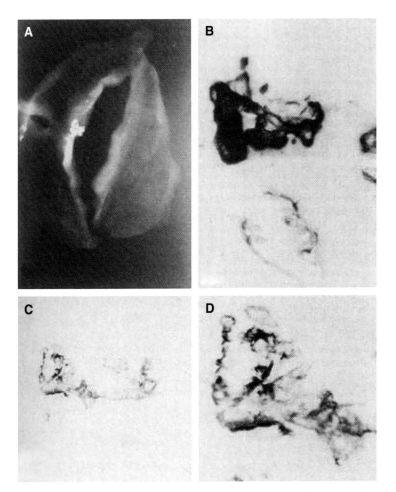

Fig. 5. Evidence of osteopontin in calcified aortic valves (*A–D*). (*From* Mohler ER III, Adam LP, McClelland P, et al. Detection of osteopontin in calcified human aortic valves. Arterioscler Thrombo Vasc Biol 1997;17(3):551; with permission.)

that the underlying mechanism of degenerative valve disease may be related to the activation of the Lrp5 receptor in the spectrum of osteoblast differentiation within human diseased valve leaflets [52]. To test this hypothesis, the author and colleagues studied degenerative mitral, calcified tricuspid, and bicuspid aortic valves to determine whether the Lrp5 signaling pathway is expressed in diseased cardiac valves [52].

The most common location of degenerative valves is the left side of the heart. Myxomatous mitral valve lesions causing mitral regurgitation are believed to be caused by progressive thickening due to activated myofibroblasts [53]. Myxomatous mitral valve prolapse in young patients is probably secondary to a genetic cause. In older patients, it is likely secondary to modifiable risk factors. Recent evidence suggests that the aortic valve develops calcification secondary to an osteoblast differentiation pathway [47]. Finally, bicuspid aortic valves develop calcification similar to that of tricuspid aortic stenosis but at an earlier age [54].

Fig. 8 demonstrates the immunohistochemistry stains for the osteoblast signaling markers Lrp5, Wnt3, and proliferating nuclear cell antigen (PCNA). Fig. 8A1, A2, B1, and B2 demonstrate a mild amount of Lrp5 and Wnt3 staining in the control valves and in the areas of hypertrophic chondrocytes in the mitral valves. Lrp5 and Wnt3 staining was increased in the calcified aortic valves (see Fig. 8A3, A4, B3, and B4). Fig. 8C3 and C4 demonstrate the presence of an increase in PCNA protein expression compared with Fig. 8C1 and C2, which demonstrate a decrease in PCNA protein staining.

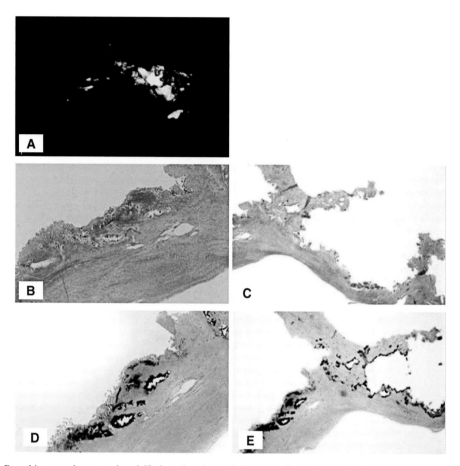

Fig. 6. Bone histomorphometery in calcified aortic valves. (*A*) Contact microradiography. (*B*) Low-power magnification of Goldner's stain for hydroxyapatite. (*C*) High-power magnification of Goldner's stain for hydroxyapatite. (*D*) Low-power magnification of von Kossa's stain for hydroxyapatite. (*E*) High-power magnification of von Kossa's stain for hydroxyapatite. (*From* Rajamannan NM, Subramaniam M, Rickard D, et al. Human aortic valve calcification is associated with an osteoblast phenotype. Circulation 2003;107(17):2182; with permission.)

This study [52] demonstrates that the Lrp5/Wnt3 signaling markers are present in the calcified aortic valve to a greater degree than in the degenerative mitral valve. These data provide the first evidence of a mechanistic pathway for the initiation of bone differentiation in degenerative valve lesions that is expressed in the mitral valve as a cartilage phenotype and in the calcified aortic valve as a bone phenotype. These results indicate that there is a continuum of an earlier stage of osteoblast bone differentiation in the mitral valves compared with the calcified aortic valves. In normal adult skeleton formation, the initiation of bone formation occurs with the development of a cartilaginous template that eventually mineralizes and forms calcified bone. Therefore, the mitral valve expresses an early cartilage

formation and the aortic valve demonstrates the mineralized osteoblast phenotype that follows the spectrum of normal skeletal bone formation. This is the first study to demonstrate the presence of chondrocytes in mitral valves and osteoblasts in aortic valves, implicating this pathologic mechanism in the development of mitral regurgitation in degenerative myxomatous mitral valves and stenosis in calcific aortic valves. These findings may be secondary to an osteoblast differentiation process that is mediated by the Lrp5/Wnt3 pathway and demonstrate an active endochondral bone formation mechanism in the development of heart valve disease. These data provide the first evidence of a mechanistic pathway for the initiation of bone differentiation in degenerative valve lesions that is expressed in the mitral

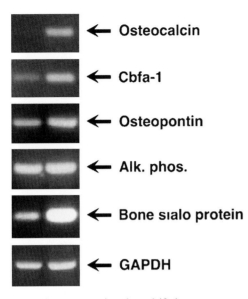

Fig. 7. Gene expression in calcified versus control aortic valves demonstrating osteoblast bone markers. Alk. Phos., alkaline phosphates. (*From* Rajamannan NM, Subramaniam M, Rickard D, et al. Human aortic valve calcification is associated with an osteoblast phenotype. Circulation 2003;107(17):2183; with permission.)

valve as a cartilage phenotype and in the calcified aortic valve as a bone phenotype [52].

Statins as a potential therapy for aortic valve stenosis

Although valve replacement is the current treatment of choice for severe critical aortic stenosis, future insights into the mechanisms of calcification and its progression may indicate a role for lipid-lowering therapy in modifying the rate of progression of stenosis. Several members of the 3-hydroxy-3-methylglutanyl (HMG) coenzyme A reductase class of drugs, long recognized as effective in lowering cholesterol levels and reducing cardiovascular risk, have recently been shown to have significant effects on cardiovascular mortality and atherosclerosis [55,56]. Whether statins influence the development of vascular and valvular calcification is not known prospectively; however, there are a growing number of studies from retrospective echocardiographic databases that have demonstrated that statin therapy may slow the progression of this disease process [20,57–60]. Fig. 9 demonstrates the potential mechanism by which lipids regulate the differentiation of the valve

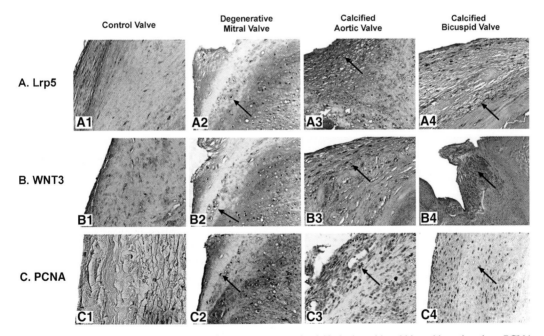

Fig. 8. Lrp5 bone signaling markers in control, myxomatous, and calcified tricuspid and bicuspid aortic valves. PCNA, proliferating nuclear cell antigen (*A–C*). (*From* Caira FC, Stock SR, Gleason TG, et al. Human degenerative valve disease is associated with up-regulation of low-density lipoprotein receptor-related protein 5 receptor-mediated bone formation. J Am Coll Cardiol 2006;47(8):1711; with permission. Copyright © 2006, American College of Cardiology Foundation.)

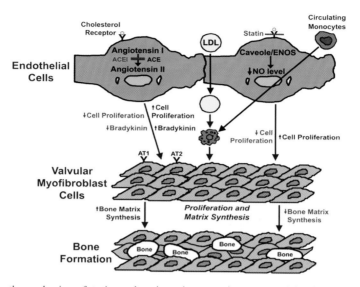

Fig. 9. Diagram for the mechanism of statins and angiotensin-converting enzyme (ACE) inhibitors in aortic valve cal-cification. AT, angiotensin; ENOS, endothelial nitric oxide synthase; NO, nitric oxide. (*From* Rajamannan NM, Otto CM. Targeted therapy to prevent progression of calcific aortic stenosis. Circulation 2004;110(11):1181; with permission.)

myofibroblast cell to a bonelike phenotype and the use of statins in the slowing of progression of this atherosclerotic disease [61]. HMG coenzyme A re-ductase inhibitors may provide an innovative ther-apeutic approach by employing lipid-lowering and possible non–lipid-lowering effects to forestall crit-ical stenosis in the aortic valve. Despite the increas-ing prevalence of this condition and the growing epidemiologic evidence demonstrating the clinical risk factors, very little is known regarding the cellu-lar mechanisms of calcific aortic stenosis. Further-more, there are no established medical treatments indicated for calcific aortic stenosis. If cholesterol is a causative risk factor, then medications may have a pivotal role in the management of aortic valve disease. The understanding of medical ther-apy in aortic valve disease may slow the progres-sion of stenosis and decrease the number of aortic valve replacements in the future.

Experimental hypercholesterolemic rabbit model demonstrates the effects of statins in atherosclerotic aortic valves

The author's laboratory has developed models of experimental hypercholesterolemia and aortic valve atherosclerosis and valve calcification. Ini-tially, the author and colleagues [39] studied an experimental rabbit model of hypercholesterol-emia for 8 weeks that produced an atherosclerotic lesion in the aortic valve. Next, they studied this

model to determine a number of different stages of valvular atherosclerosis and eventual minerali-zation in these tissues. The following stage investi-gated whether hypercholesterolemia causes an atherosclerotic proliferative valve lesion associ-ated with the expression of an osteoblast-like phe-notype [40]. During this study, the author and colleagues also tested whether atorvastatin would inhibit this process in the aortic valve.

Fig. 10A1 and B1 demonstrate that the normal aortic valve surface from control animals ap-peared thin and intact, with a smooth endothelial cell layer covering the entire surface and a thin collagen layer in the spongiosa layer of the valve, as demonstrated by hematoxylin-eosin stain and Masson trichrome stain. There were no macro-phages or proliferation in the aortic valves of nor-mal control rabbits (see Fig. 10C1 and D1). In contrast, the aortic valves from the hyperchol-esterolemic animals demonstrated fatty plaque for-mation with scant accumulation of basophilic material. Foam cells converged to form a large lipid-laden lesion on the aortic endocardial sur-face of the valve leaflets (see Fig. 10A2). There was also an increase in the blue collagen trichrome stain in the hypercholesterolemic aortic valves (Fig. 10B2). The endothelial layer on the valve surface appeared disrupted by infiltration of extracellular lipid deposits, myofibroblast cells, and foam cells, which stain positive for macro-phages (RAM 11) (see Fig. 10C2). These lesions

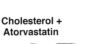

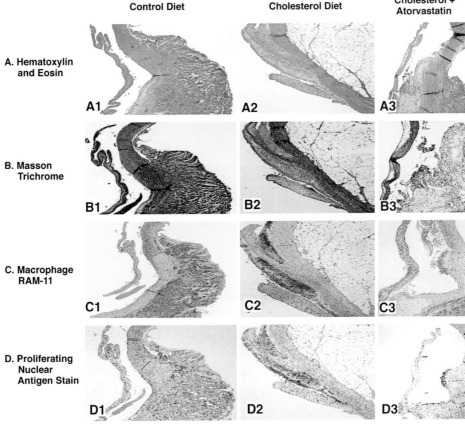

Fig. 10. Atorvastatin attenuates atherosclerosis in the rabbit aortic valve. (*A*) Hematoxylin-eosin stain. (*B*) Masson tri-chrome stain. (*C*) Macrophage: RAM-11 stain. (*D*) Proliferating nuclear cell antigen stain. (*From* Rajamannan NM, Subramaniam M, Springett M, et al. Atorvastatin inhibits hypercholesterolemia-induced cellular proliferation and bone matrix production in the rabbit aortic valve. Circulation 2002;105(22):2662; with permission.)

developed primarily at the base of the leaflets and decreased in extent toward the leaflet tips. The hy-percholesterolemic aortic valves also demon-strated a marked increase in myofibroblast PCNA staining along the base of the aortic valve (see Fig. 10D2). The atorvastatin-treated rabbits demonstrated a marked decrease in the amount of atherosclerotic plaque burden, macrophage in-filtration, and proliferation (see Fig. 10A3, B3, C3, and D3), and these changes were most pro-nounced at the base of the leaflets. This study is the first experimental study to test the effect of a statin on atherosclerosis and cell proliferation on the aortic valve lesion.

The author and colleagues' [62] next study was to determine whether calcification was developing in the aortic valve. To test this hypothesis, they tested the rabbit model for 3 months instead of

2 months to allow the valves to mineralize. Fur-thermore, identification of the intermediate signal-ing steps between lipid accumulation, cellular proliferation, and calcification have not been clearly established. Studying the signaling path-ways in disease processes helps to develop future targeted therapies for aortic stenosis. The normal aortic valve surface from control animals ap-peared thin and intact, with a smooth endothelial cell layer covering the entire surface and a thin collagen layer within the spongiosa. There was lit-tle to no endothelial nitric oxide synthase (eNOS) immunostaining present in the endothelium (Fig. 11A1). In contrast, the aortic valves from the hypercholesterolemic animals demonstrated an atherosclerotic lesion along the aortic surface that was identifiable by light microscopy (see Fig. 11A2). Again, there was no evidence of

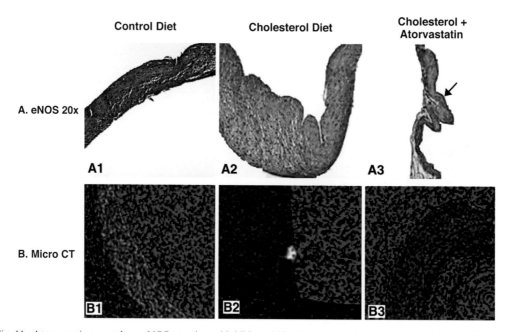

Fig. 11. Atorvastatin upregulates eNOS protein and inhibits calcification in the rabbit aortic valve. (*A*) eNOS immuno-histochemistry. (*B*) Masson trichrome stain. (*From* Rajamannan NM, Subramaniam M, Stock SR, et al. Atorvastatin inhibits calcification and enhances nitric oxide synthase production in the hypercholesterolaemic aortic valve. Heart 2005;91(6):806–10; with permission.)

eNOS immunostaining along the surface of the aortic valve. The atorvastatin-treated rabbits demonstrated a marked decrease in the amount of atherosclerotic plaque burden, with a positive immunostain for eNOS in the endothelial layer of the aortic valve (see arrow in Fig. 11A3). MicroCT was used to evaluate the development of calcification in valve leaflets and the aorta in each of the treatment groups. Control aortic valves and aortas demonstrated little-to-no mineralization (see Fig. 11B1). The hypercholesterolemic aortic valves and aortas appeared to be in early stages of calcification (see Fig. 11B2). In the group given cholesterol plus atorvastatin, the aortic valves and aortas could not be distinguished from those of the controls (see Fig. 11B1 and B3).

Nitric oxide is generated in vascular endothelial cells by eNOS and is responsible for endothelial-dependent vasorelaxation, inhibition of smooth muscle cell proliferation, and decreased synthesis of extracellular matrix proteins. Nitric oxide is a key regulator of normal endothelial function in the vasculature. Structurally, an endothelial layer lines the aortic valve leaflet. Charest and colleagues [63] also demonstrated that eNOS is expressed in human calcified aortic valves. These data provide the initial evidence

that eNOS produced in the valve endothelium has a role in the physiologic cellular regulation of this tissue similar to its role in vascular endothelium. This inactivation of eNOS leads to a decrease in the availability of nitric oxide. This inhibitory action of hypercholesterolemia on eNOS activity may play a critical role in the development of mineralization of the atherosclerotic aortic valve over time, which can be reversed with statin therapy.

Finally, the author and colleagues [50] tested the experimental hypercholesterolemic rabbit model for 6 months to determine whether the valves develop extensive mineralization and whether an osteoblast signaling pathway is present in the calcifying aortic valve. In this study, they tested for the regulation of the Lrp5 receptor in the presence of cholesterol and statin therapy. LDL receptors are critical in the uptake, processing, and cellular metabolism of cholesterol. In this study, the Watanabe rabbit, with a naturally occurring genetic LDL receptor mutation, serves as an important genetic model for the inheritable cholesterol disease FH. Studies have demonstrated that FH patients have extensive calcification in their vasculature and aortic valves [58]. In the author and colleagues' most recent experimental hypercholesterolemia experiment in the naturally occurring LDL knockout Watanabe rabbit (a genetic model for FH), they demonstrated that osteoblast-like calcification develops in the rabbit aortic valves after 6 months, which is regulated by LRP5 and modified by atorvastatin treatment [50]. These studies provide further evidence toward the multifactorial cellular pathways involved in aortic valve calcification by way of experimental hypercholesterolemia.

The hypercholesterolemic aortic valves stained with hematoxylin-eosin and Masson trichrome stain shown in Fig. 12A2, B2, and C2 demonstrate an increase in leaflet thickness that begins at the base of the aortic valve leaflet and extends along the valve leaflet from the attachment to the aorta, with an increase in the Lrp5 red staining receptors. There is a marked increase in cellularity and collagen staining in the blue Masson trichrome throughout the leaflet lesion. The aortic valve surface from control animals appeared normal, thin, and intact, with a smooth endothelial cell layer covering the entire surface and a thin collagen layer in the spongiosa of the valve (see Fig. 12A1, B1, and C1). Abnormal leaflet thicknesses did not develop when cholesterol-fed rabbits received atorvastatin with attenuation of the Lrp5 staining (see Fig. 12A3, B3, and C3).

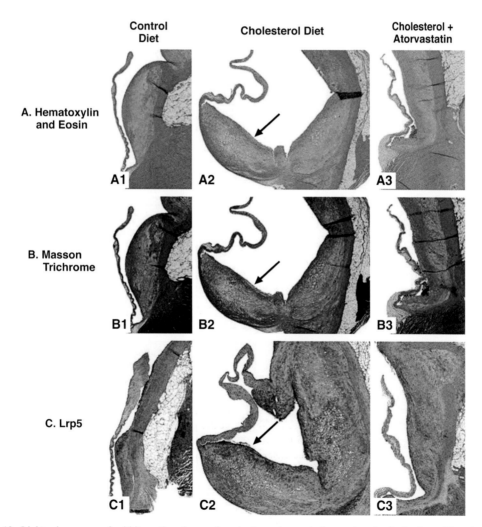

Fig. 12. Light microscopy of rabbit aortic valves and aorta. In each panel, the aortic valve leaflet is positioned on the left, with the aorta on the right. Arrows point to aortic valve. (All frames ×12.5 magnification.) (*A*) Hematoxylin-eosin stain. (*B*) Masson trichrome stain. (*C*) Lrp5 receptor immunostain.

In this study, the author and colleagues [50] demonstrated that calcification of the aortic valve leaflets develops within the valve similar to skeletal bone formation and that this mineralization occurs with the up-regulation of Lrp5 receptors and bone formation in the cholesterol-treated rabbit valve and a decrease in the receptor and bone formation with the atorvastatin treatment. Lrp5 is a critical LDL coreceptor important in the differentiation of osteoblast cells in skeletal bone formation [48,49]. The naturally occurring LDL receptor defect in Watanabe rabbits has made this species a parallel model to FH patients who have mutations in the LDL receptor [64]. Electron beam CT studies demonstrate that FH patients have accelerated vascular and valvular atherosclerosis and calcification [65]. This study extends the author and colleagues' original experimental studies

demonstrating atherosclerosis and cell proliferation in a short-term, cholesterol-feeding rabbit model to demonstrate the findings in a long-term, lower concentration of cholesterol feeding.

Retrospective studies evaluating statins in aortic valve disease

Currently, there are six retrospective studies in echocardiographic and electron beam CT databases that demonstrate the efficacy of statin and angiotensin-converting enzyme (ACE) inhibitor therapy in the treatment of aortic valve stenosis (Table 2) [20,57–60,66,67]. These studies demonstrate that the progression of aortic stenosis is slowed in patients who have aortic valve disease and are already on statin therapy and ACE inhibitors as shown by echocardiographic parameters

Table 2
Nonrandomized retrospective studies of medical therapy to prevent progression of calcific aortic stenosis

Study	N	Mean age (% men)	Mean follow-up interval	Study group	Change	P
BCT calcium						
Pohle et al, 2001 [58]	104	65 y (86%)	1.25 y	LDL ≤130 mg/dL	9 ± 22%[a]	≤.001
				LDL >130 mg/dL	43 ± 44%[a]	
Shavelle et al, 2002 [59]	65	67 y	2.5 y	Statin therapy (43%)	12.1%[a]	.006
				No statin therapy	32%[a]	
Echocardiography						
Aronow et al, 2001 [20]	180	82 y (31%)	2.8 y	LDL ≥125 mg/dL not on statin	6.3 ± 1.4[b]	<.0001
				LDL ≥125 mg/dL on statin	3.4 ± 1.0[b]	
				LDL <125 mg/dL not on statin	3.1 ± 1.1[b]	
Novaro et al, 2001 [60]	174	68 y (44%)	1.8 y	Statin therapy (33%)	0.06 ± 0.16[c]	.03
				No Statin therapy	0.11 ± 0.18[c]	
Bellamy et al, 2002 [57]	156	77 y (58%)	3.7 y	Statin therapy (24%)	0.04 ± 0.15[c]	.04
				No statin therapy	0.09 ± 0.17[c]	
Rosenhek et al, 2004 [66]	211	70 y	2.0 y	Statin therapy	0.10 ± 0.41[d]	.0001
				No statin therapy	0.39 ± 0.42[d]	
				ACE inhibitor	0.29 ± 0.44[d]	
				No ACE inhibitor	0.35 ± 0.44[d]	.29

Abbreviation: EBCT, electron beam CT.
[a] Percentage increase in valve calcium per year.
[b] Increase in peak gradient (mm Hg/y).
[c] Decrease in value area (cm^2/y).
[d] Increase in aortic velocity (m/s/y).
Data from Rajamannan, NM, Otto CM. Targeted therapy to prevent progression of calcific aortic stenosis. Circulation 2004;110(10):1181.

and electron beam CT. The patients who had aortic stenosis in these databases were already taking medications targeting LDL and hypertension. Furthermore, these studies demonstrate the potential effect of slowing the progression of their aortic stenosis with these medications.

Another important medication for the treatment of atherosclerosis is ACE inhibitors. These medications interfere with the rennin-angiotensin system and exert beneficial effects on vascular tissues, including inhibition of cellular proliferation and matrix productions. ACE inhibitors reduced atherogenesis in experimental models by inhibiting the conversion of inactive angiotensin I to active angiotensin II and by decreasing bradykinin levels, resulting in improved endothelial function. O'Brien and colleagues [68] showed the presence of ACE in tissues from patients who had aortic valve disease. Fig. 13 demonstrates the positive immunohistochemistry for ACE and the colocalization with LDL in these tissues [68].

Rosenhek and colleagues [66] tested for the effects of the potential for ACE inhibitor therapy on aortic valve stenosis progression. These investigators found no significant difference in disease progression in patients taking ACE inhibitor therapy compared with those not taking an ACE inhibitor, despite careful consideration of the effects of coexisting hypertension. Although the data in this study demonstrate that the effect of ACE inhibitors on the progression of aortic stenosis is negative, there is the potential for targeting this signaling pathway in the future. O'Brien and colleagues' [68] data indicate the potential for this pathway. Prospective studies for ACE inhibitor therapy are necessary for proper evaluation and timing using this treatment in this patient population. It may require an earlier timing for these ACE inhibitors in aortic valve sclerosis as opposed to aortic stenosis [66].

Prospective studies for statins and aortic valve disease

The first randomized prospective study testing the effects of statins in aortic valve disease was published in 2005 [69]. In this double-blind placebo-controlled trial, patients who had calcific aortic stenosis were randomly assigned to receive 80 mg of atorvastatin daily or a matched placebo. Aortic valve stenosis and calcification were assessed with the use of Doppler echocardiography and helical CT, respectively. The primary end

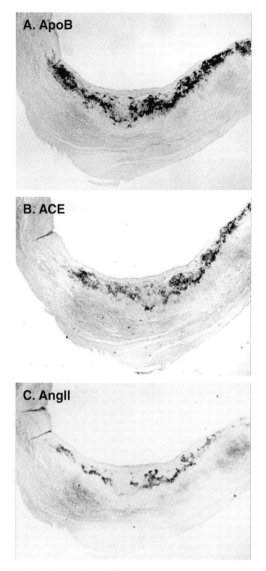

Fig. 13. Association of ACE with LDL in aortic valvular lesions and in human plasma (*A–C*). (*From* O'Brien KD, Shavelle DM, Caulfield MT, et al. Association of angiotensin-converting enzyme with low-density lipoprotein in aortic valvular lesions and in human plasma. Circulation 2002;106(17):2222; with permission.)

points were change in aortic-jet velocity and aortic-valve calcium score. Seventy-seven patients were assigned to atorvastatin and 78 to placebo, with a median follow-up of 25 months. Serum LDL cholesterol concentrations remained at 130 $\pm$ 30 mg/dL in the placebo group and fell to 63 $\pm$ 23 mg/dL in the atorvastatin group. Increases in aortic-jet velocity were 0.199 $\pm$ 0.210 m/sec per year in the atorvastatin group and 0.203 ± 0.208 m/sec per year in the placebo group. Progression in valvular calcification was 22.3 ± 21.0% per year in the atorvastatin group and 21.7 ± 19.8% per year in the placebo group.

The Scottish aortic stenosis and lipid lowering therapy, impact on regression (SALTIRE) investigators concluded that intensive lipid-lowering therapy does not halt the progression of calcific aortic stenosis or induce its regression. This study, published in the *New England Journal of Medicine*, was a landmark study in the field of statin therapy for aortic valve disease. The major difficulty with the study design is that the patients treated with atorvastatin received the therapy too late in the course of the disease process. In view of the experimental data, the earlier in the disease process the statin therapy is initiated, the better the potential for slowing the progression of this disease.

Currently, there are three other prospective clinical trials testing the effects of statins in aortic valve disease: Aortic Stenosis Progression Observation Measuring Effects of Rosuvastatin (Canada); Simvastatin and the Ezetimibe in Aortic Stenosis (Europe) [70]; and Stop Aortic Stenosis (Cleveland Clinic, Cleveland, Ohio). The Rousvastatin Affecting Aortic Valve Endothelium (RAAVE) trial suggested that earlier treatment with statin is more efficacious in the prevention of progression of aortic valve stenosis than late treatment, similar to the effects of statins in the regression of vascular atherosclerosis [71].

In the RAAVE trial [72], prospective treatment of aortic stenosis with Rosuvastatin targeting serum LDL slowed the progression of echocardiographic hemodynamic measurements and improved inflammatory biomarkers, providing the first clinical evidence for targeted therapy in patients who have asymptomatic aortic stenosis. The study's aim was to assess rosuvastatin on the hemodynamic progression and inflammatory markers of aortic stenosis by treating LDL for 1 year in patients who have aortic stenosis according to the National Cholesterol Education Program (NCEP)-ATPIII guidelines. The RAAVE investigators performed an open-label, prospective study evaluating 118 consecutive patients who had asymptomatic moderate aortic stenosis (aged 73.5 ± 8.8 years; 56 men and 62 women), with and without rosuvastatin according to the NCEP-ATPIII guidelines. Echocardiographic and serum markers for (hs)C-reactive protein, interleukin-6, and CD40 were measured at baseline and every 6 months for 1 year.

Sixty-five patients (55.1%) who had elevated LDL (162 ± 35.7 mg/dL), aortic valve velocity (3.62 ± 0.63 m/s), and aortic valve area (1.11 ± 0.38 cm²) received rosuvastatin (20 mg/d); 53 patients (44.9%) who had normal LDL (108.4 ± 20.9 mg/dL), aortic valve velocity (3.64 ± 0.61 m/s), and aortic valve area (1.10 ± 0.37 cm²) received no statin.

During a mean follow-up of 53 ± 3.2 weeks, the decrease in aortic valve area was 0.11 ± 0.18 cm² in the nonstatin group versus 0.04 ± 0.13 cm² in the statin treatment group ($P = .059$). The change in peak aortic valve velocity was 0.18 ± 0.26 m/s in the statin treatment group versus 0.04 ± 0.29 m/s in the nonstatin group ($P = .016$). There was statistical improvement in all serum markers in the statin group. Prospective treatment of moderate aortic stenosis with rosuvastatin targeting serum LDL slowed progression of aortic valve peak velocity and improved inflammatory biomarkers, showing the first clinical evidence for targeted therapy in asymptomatic moderate-to-severe aortic stenosis [72].

Summary

Our understanding of aortic valve disease has evolved in the past decade from a degenerative process to an active biologic disease. Results of the SALTIRE trial demonstrate that future clinical trials for this disease process are important and that timing of the initiation of therapy is critical in the potential treatment of this disease. The results of this trial have provided important guidelines for enrollment criteria and baseline characteristics for initiation of future aortic valve trials. Aortic valve disease, although it has a similar atherosclerotic pathogenesis, is a different disease process in terms of bone calcification. The timing of statin therapy to slow the progression of bone formation in these lesions will dictate the future of medical therapy for these patients. The SALTIRE trial has clearly proved this important effect with the late initiation of treatment in this clinical trial. Understanding of the biology of the valve lesion will play an important role in the understanding of this disease and the future treatment options for these patients.

References

[1] Society of Thoracic Surgeons. Adult cardiac national database: spring 2004 executive summary. Available at: www.sts.org. Accessed June 23, 2006.

[2] Bonow RO, Carabello B, de Leon AC Jr, et al. Guidelines for the management of patients with valvular heart disease: executive summary. A report of the American College of Cardiology/American Heart Association Task Force on Practice Guidelines (Committee on Management of Patients with Valvular Heart Disease). Circulation 1998;98(18):1949–84.

[3] Stokes W. The diseases of the heart and aorta. Dublin, Ireland: Hodges & Smith; 1845.

[4] Rye K-A, Wee K, Curtiss LK, et al. Apolipoprotein A-II inhibits high density lipoprotein remodeling and lipid-poor apolipoprotein A-I formation. J Biol Chem 2003;278(25):22530–6.

[5] Tabas I. Consequences of cellular cholesterol accumulation: basic concepts and physiological implications. J Clin Invest 2002;110(7):905–11.

[6] Thukkani AK, McHowat J, Hsu FF, et al. Identification of alpha-chloro fatty aldehydes and unsaturated lysophosphatidylcholine molecular species in human atherosclerotic lesions. Circulation 2003; 108(25):3128–33.

[7] Koh KP, Wang Y, Yi T, et al. T cell-mediated vascular dysfunction of human allografts results from IFN-{gamma} dysregulation of NO synthase. J Clin Invest 2004;114(6):846–56.

[8] Cheitlin M, Armstrong W, Aurigemma G, et al. ACC/AHA/ASE 2003 guideline update for the clinical application of echocardiography: summary article: a report of the American College of Cardiology/ American Heart Association Task Force on Practice Guidelines (ACC/AHA/ASE Committee to Update the 1997 Guidelines for the Clinical Application of Echocardiography). J Am Soc Echocardiogr 2003; 16(10):1091–110.

[9] Charo IF, Taubman MB. Chemokines in the pathogenesis of vascular disease. Circ Res 2004;95(9): 858–66.

[10] Adams LD, Geary RL, McManus B, et al. A comparison of aorta and vena cava medial message expression by cDNA array analysis identifies a set of 68 consistently differentially expressed genes, all in aortic media. Circ Res 2000;87(7):623–31.

[11] Towler DA, Bidder M, Latifi T, et al. Diet-induced diabetes activates an osteogenic gene regulatory program in the aortas of low density lipoprotein receptor-deficient mice. J Biol Chem 1998;273(46): 30427–34.

[12] Deutscher S, Rockette HE, Krishnaswami V. Diabetes and hypercholesterolemia among patients with calcific aortic stenosis. J Chronic Dis 1984;37(5): 407–15.

[13] Aronow WS, Schwartz KS, Koenigsberg M. Correlation of serum lipids, calcium, and phosphorus, diabetes mellitus and history of systemic hypertension with presence or absence of calcified or thickened aortic cusps or root in elderly patients. Am J Cardiol 1987;59(9):998–9.

[14] Mohler ER, Sheridan MJ, Nichols R, et al. Development and progression of aortic valve stenosis:

atherosclerosis risk factors—a causal relationship? A clinical morphologic study. Clin Cardiol 1991; 14(12):995–9.

[15] Lindroos M, Kupari M, Valvanne J, et al. Factors associated with calcific aortic valve degeneration in the elderly. Eur Heart J 1994;15(7):865–70.

[16] Boon A, Cheriex E, Lodder J, et al. Cardiac valve calcification: characteristics of patients with calcification of the mitral annulus or aortic valve. Heart 1997;78(5):472–4.

[17] Stewart BF, Siscovick D, Lind BK, et al. Clinical factors associated with calcific aortic valve disease. Cardiovascular Health Study. J Am Coll Cardiol 1997;29(3):630–4.

[18] Wilmshurst PT, Stevenson RN, Griffiths H, et al. A case-control investigation of the relation between hyperlipidaemia and calcific aortic valve stenosis. Heart 1997;78(5):475–9.

[19] Chan KL, Ghani M, Woodend K, et al. Case-controlled study to assess risk factors for aortic stenosis in congenitally bicuspid aortic valve. Am J Cardiol 2001;88(6):690–3.

[20] Aronow WS, Ahn C, Kronzon I, et al. Association of coronary risk factors and use of statins with progression of mild valvular aortic stenosis in older persons. Am J Cardiol 2001;88(6):693–5.

[21] Chui MC, Newby DE, Panarelli M, et al. Association between calcific aortic stenosis and hypercholesterolemia: is there a need for a randomized controlled trial of cholesterol-lowering therapy? Clin Cardiol 2001;24(1):52–5.

[22] Peltier M, Trojette F, Sarano ME, et al. Relation between cardiovascular risk factors and nonrheumatic severe calcific aortic stenosis among patients with a three-cuspid aortic valve. Am J Cardiol 2003; 91(1):97–9.

[23] Whyte HM. The relative importance of the major risk factors in atherosclerotic and other diseases. Aust N Z J Med 1976;6(5):387–93.

[24] Wilson PW, Castelli WP, et al. Coronary risk prediction in adults (the Framingham Heart Study). Am J Cardiol 1987;59(14):91G–4G.

[25] D'Agostino RB, Kannel WB, Belanger AJ, et al. Trends in CHD and risk factors at age 55–64 in the Framingham Study. Int J Epidemiol 1989;18 (3, Suppl 1):S67–72.

[26] Olsson M, Thyberg J, Nilsson J. Presence of oxidized low density lipoprotein in nonrheumatic stenotic aortic valves. Arterioscler Thromb Vasc Biol 1999; 19(5):1218–22.

[27] O'Brien KD, Reichenbach DD, Marcovina SM, et al. Apolipoproteins B, (a), and E accumulate in the morphologically early lesion of 'degenerative' valvular aortic stenosis. Arterioscler Thromb Vasc Biol 1996;16(4):523–32.

[28] Hsu SY, Hung KC, Chang SH, et al. C-reactive protein in predicting coronary artery disease in subjects with aortic valve sclerosis before diagnostic coronary angiography. Am J Med Sci 2006;331(5):264–9.

[29] Sanchez PL, Santos JL, Kaski JC, et al. Relation of circulating C-reactive protein to progression of aortic valve stenosis. Am J Cardiol 2006;97(1):90–3.

[30] Skowasch D, Schrempf S, Preusse CJ, et al. Tissue resident C reactive protein in degenerative aortic valves: correlation with serum C reactive protein concentrations and modification by statins. Heart 2006;92(4):495–8.

[31] Jian B, Narula N, Li QY, et al. Progression of aortic valve stenosis: TGF-beta1 is present in calcified aortic valve cusps and promotes aortic valve interstitial cell calcification via apoptosis. Ann Thorac Surg 2003;75(2):457–65 [discussion: 65–6].

[32] Narine K, DeWever O, Cathenis K, et al. Transforming growth factor-beta-induced transition of fibroblasts: a model for myofibroblast procurement in tissue valve engineering. J Heart Valve Dis 2004; 13(2):281–9 [discussion: 9].

[33] Sprecher DL, Schaefer EJ, Kent KM, et al. Cardiovascular features of homozygous familial hypercholesterolemia: analysis of 16 patients. Am J Cardiol 1984;54(1):20–30.

[34] Rajamannan NM, Edwards WD, Spelsberg TC. Hypercholesterolemic aortic-valve disease. N Engl J Med 2003;349(7):717–8.

[35] Buja LM, Kovanen PT, Bilheimer DW. Cellular pathology of homozygous familial hypercholesterolemia. Am J Pathol 1979;97(2):327–57.

[36] Kawaguchi A, Miyatake K, Yutani C, et al. Characteristic cardiovascular manifestation in homozygous and heterozygous familial hypercholesterolemia. Am Heart J 1999;137(3):410–8.

[37] Kawaguchi A, Yutani C, Yamamoto A. Hypercholesterolemic valvulopathy: an aspect of malignant atherosclerosis. Ther Apher Dial 2003;7(4): 439–43.

[38] Drolet MC, Arsenault M, Couet J. Experimental aortic valve stenosis in rabbits. J Am Coll Cardiol 2003;41(7):1211–7.

[39] Rajamannan NM, Sangiorgi G, Springett M, et al. Experimental hypercholesterolemia induces apoptosis in the aortic valve. J Heart Valve Dis 2001;10(3): 371–4.

[40] Rajamannan NM, Subramaniam M, Springett M, et al. Atorvastatin inhibits hypercholesterolemia-induced cellular proliferation and bone matrix production in the rabbit aortic valve. Circulation 2002; 105(22):2260–5.

[41] Sarphie TG. A cytochemical study of the surface properties of aortic and mitral valve endothelium from hypercholesterolemic rabbits. Exp Mol Pathol 1986;44(3):281–96.

[42] Becker CR, Majeed A, Crispin A, et al. CT measurement of coronary calcium mass: impact on global cardiac risk assessment. Eur Radiol 2005;15(1): 96–101.

[43] Rosenhek R, Binder T, Porenta G, et al. Predictors of outcome in severe, asymptomatic aortic stenosis. N Engl J Med 2000;343(9):611–7.

[44] Mohler ER III, Gannon F, Reynolds C, et al. Bone formation and inflammation in cardiac valves. Circulation 2001;103(11):1522–8.

[45] Mohler ER III, Adam LP, McClelland P, et al. Detection of osteopontin in calcified human aortic valves. Arterioscler Thromb Vasc Biol 1997;17(3): 547–52.

[46] O'Brien KD, Kuusisto J, Reichenbach DD, et al. Osteopontin is expressed in human aortic valvular lesions. Circulation 1995;92(8):2163–8.

[47] Rajamannan NM, Subramaniam M, Rickard D, et al. Human aortic valve calcification is associated with an osteoblast phenotype. Circulation 2003; 107(17):2181–4.

[48] Gong Y, Slee RB, Fukai N, et al. LDL receptor-related protein 5 (LRP5) affects bone accrual and eye development. Cell 2001;107(4):513–23.

[49] Little RD, Carulli JP, Del Mastro RG, et al. A mutation in the LDL receptor-related protein 5 gene results in the autosomal dominant high-bone-mass trait. Am J Hum Genet 2002;70(1):11–9.

[50] Rajamannan NM, Subramaniam M, Caira FC, et al. Atorvastatin inhibits hypercholesterolemia-induced calcification in the aortic valves via the Lrp5 receptor pathway. Circulation 2005;112(Suppl 9):1229–34.

[51] Shao JS, Cheng SL, Pingsterhaus JM, et al. Msx2 promotes cardiovascular calcification by activating paracrine Wnt signals. J Clin Invest 2005;115(5): 1210–20.

[52] Caira FC, Stock SR, Gleason TG, et al. Human degenerative valve disease is associated with up-regulation of low-density lipoprotein receptor-related protein 5 receptor-mediated bone formation. J Am Coll Cardiol 2006;47(8):1707–12.

[53] Rabkin E, Aikawa M, Stone JR, et al. Activated interstitial myofibroblasts express catabolic enzymes and mediate matrix remodeling in myxomatous heart valves. Circulation 2001;104(21):2525–32.

[54] Roberts WC, Ko JM. Frequency by decades of unicuspid, bicuspid, and tricuspid aortic valves in adults having isolated aortic valve replacement for aortic stenosis, with or without associated aortic regurgitation. Circulation 2005;111(7):920–5.

[55] Randomised trial of cholesterol lowering in 4444 patients with coronary heart disease: the Scandinavian Simvastatin Survival Study (4S). Lancet 1994; 344(8934):1383–9.

[56] Shepherd J, Cobbe SM, Ford I, et al. Prevention of coronary heart disease with pravastatin in men with hypercholesterolemia. West of Scotland Coronary Prevention Study Group. N Engl J Med 1995; 333(20):1301–7.

[57] Bellamy MF, Pellikka PA, Klarich KW, et al. Association of cholesterol levels, hydroxymethylglutaryl coenzyme-A reductase inhibitor treatment, and progression of aortic stenosis in the community [comment]. J Am Coll Cardiol 2002;40(10):1723–30.

[58] Pohle K, Maffert R, Ropers D, et al. Progression of aortic valve calcification: association with coronary

atherosclerosis and cardiovascular risk factors. Circulation 2001;104(16):1927–32.

[59] Shavelle DM, Takasu J, Budoff MJ, et al. HMG CoA reductase inhibitor (statin) and aortic valve calcium. Lancet 2002;359(9312):1125–6.

[60] Novaro GM, Tiong IY, Pearce GL, et al. Effect of hydroxymethylglutaryl coenzyme a reductase inhibitors on the progression of calcific aortic stenosis. Circulation 2001;104(18):2205–9.

[61] Rajamannan NM, Otto CM. Targeted therapy to prevent progression of calcific aortic stenosis. Circulation 2004;110(10):1180–2.

[62] Rajamannan NM, Subramaniam M, Stock SR, et al. Atorvastatin inhibits calcification and enhances nitric oxide synthase production in the hypercholesterolaemic aortic valve. Heart 2005;91(6):806–10.

[63] Charest A, Pepin A, Shetty R, et al. Distribution of SPARC during neovascularization of degenerative aortic stenosis. Heart 2006;92(12):1844–9.

[64] Aliev G, Burnstock G. Watanabe rabbits with heritable hypercholesterolaemia: a model of atherosclerosis. Histol Histopathol 1998;13(3):797–817.

[65] Hoeg JM, Feuerstein IM, Tucker EE. Detection and quantitation of calcific atherosclerosis by ultrafast computed tomography in children and young adults with homozygous familial hypercholesterolemia. Arterioscler Thromb 1994;14(7):1066–74.

[66] Rosenhek R, Rader F, Loho N, et al. Statins but not angiotensin-converting enzyme inhibitors delay progression of aortic stenosis. Circulation 2004;110(10): 1291–5.

[67] O'Brien KD, Zhao XQ, Shavelle DM, et al. Hemodynamic effects of the angiotensin-converting enzyme inhibitor, ramipril, in patients with mild to moderate aortic stenosis and preserved left ventricular function. J Investig Med 2004;52(3): 185–91.

[68] O'Brien KD, Shavelle DM, Caulfield MT, et al. Association of angiotensin-converting enzyme with low-density lipoprotein in aortic valvular lesions and in human plasma. Circulation 2002;106(17): 2224–30.

[69] Cowell SJ, Newby DE, Prescott RJ, et al. A randomized trial of intensive lipid-lowering therapy in calcific aortic stenosis. N Engl J Med 2005;352(23): 2389–97.

[70] Rossebo A, Pedersen T, Skjaerpe T, et al. Design of the Simvastatin and Ezetimide in Aortic Stenosis (SEAS) study. Atherosclerosis 2003;170(Suppl 4): 253 [abstract].

[71] Nissen SE, Nicholls SJ, Sipahi I, et al. Effect of very high-intensity statin therapy on regression of coronary atherosclerosis: the ASTEROID trial. JAMA 2006;295(13):1556–65.

[72] Moura LM, Ramos SF, Zamorano JL, et al. Rousvastatin Affecting Aortic Valve Endothelium (RAAVE) to slow the progression of aortic stenosis. Circulation 2005;3224:II688.

[73] Hoagland PM, Cook EF, Flatley M, et al. Case-control analysis of risk factors for presence of aortic stenosis in adults (age 50 years or older). Am J Cardiol 1985;55(6):744–7.

ELSEVIER
SAUNDERS

Heart Failure Clin 2 (2006) 415–424

HEART
FAILURE
CLINICS

Cellular and Molecular Basis of Remodeling in Valvular Heart Diseases

Jeffrey S. Borer, MD*, Edmund McM. Herrold, MD, PhD,
John N. Carter, PhD, Daniel F. Catanzaro, PhD,
Phyllis G. Supino, EdD

*The Howard Gilman Institute for Valvular Heart Diseases, Weill Medical College of Cornell University,
New York, NY, USA*

Valvular heart diseases are disorders of the valvular structures that control blood flow into and out of the four cardiac chambers. When valves fail to open or close normally (ie, when they are stenotic or regurgitant), abnormal pressure or volume loads are imposed on the ventricular and atrial myocardium, leading to cellular and molecular adaptations that ultimately can result in heart failure and premature death.

Dr. Borer is the Gladys and Roland Harriman Professor of Cardiovascular Medicine and is supported in part by an endowment from the Gladys and Roland Harriman Foundation, New York, NY. This work also was supported by grants from the National Heart, Lung, and Blood Institute, Bethesda, MD (RO1-HL-26504, J. Borer, P.I.); The Howard Gilman Foundation, New York, NY; The Schiavone Family Foundation, White House Station, NJ; The Charles and Jean Brunie Foundation, Bronxville, NY; The David Margolis Foundation, New York, NY; The American Cardiovascular Research Foundation, New York, NY; The Irving A. Hansen Foundation, New York, NY; The Mary A.H. Rumsey Foundation, New York, NY; The Messinger Family Foundation, New York, NY; The Daniel and Elaine Sargent Charitable Trust, New York, NY; The A.C. Israel Foundation, Greenwich, CT; and by much appreciated gifts from Donna and William Acquavella, New York, NY; Maryjane Voute Arrigoni and the late William Voute, Bronxville, NY; Gerald Tanenbaum, New York, NY; and Stephen and Suzanne Weiss, Greenwich, CT.

* Corresponding author. New York-Presbyterian Hospital, New York Weill Cornell Center, 525 East 68th Street, New York, NY 10021.

E-mail address: canadad45@aol.com (J.S. Borer).

The understanding of these fundamental adaptations can be very useful. First, such knowledge can serve as a basis for the development of novel therapies to retard the natural progression of myocardial dysfunction. Second, clarification of the cellular and molecular adaptations can be expected to enable identification of biomarkers that may improve prognostication, helping to facilitate optimal selection among currently available therapies and to define management strategies.

Since the dawn of modern molecular biology two decades ago, substantial efforts have been made to elucidate the myocardial responses to the mechanical loads of valvular diseases. From these efforts, it has become clear that at the cellular and molecular levels, stenotic and regurgitant diseases are pathophysiologically distinct, and diseases of ventricular inflow valves result in myocardial responses that differ from those of ventricular outflow valves.

Additionally, in valve diseases (as in other myocardial disorders) multiple cell types, most prominently the cardiomyocyte and the cardiac fibroblast as well as endothelial cells and resident formed blood elements, are importantly involved in myocardial pathophysiological responses. The specific cellular response varies with the diseased valve.

Comprehensive review of the extensive myocardial changes that occur in all major valve diseases is beyond the scope of this article. The authors' primary focus is the disordered biology of the cardiac fibroblast and extracellular matrix (ECM) in aortic regurgitation (AR) as an example of the knowledge emerging in the area of valvular diseases. Selected data relating to the cardiomyocyte in AR, aortic stenosis (AS), and mitral regurgitation (MR), and comparative information about the ECM in AS, is provided to emphasize the important differences among these diseases.

Myocardial "remodeling": fundamental concepts

The heart has a considerable capacity to alter size, shape, and cell/molecular biology in response to hemodynamic and other environmental changes and, in so doing, to maintain external work performance at clinically acceptable levels [1]. Indeed, recent evidence of cardiac specific stem cells [2], which reside in the myocardium and presumably are capable of differentiating via an adaptive genetic program when appropriately signaled, has altered conventional beliefs about the limited capacity for adaptation of the "fully differentiated" cardiomyocyte. Moreover, even differentiated cardiomyocytes may be capable of hyperplasia in certain circumstances [3]. Perhaps more importantly, the cardiomyocyte is capable of cellular hypertrophy resulting from net synthesis or subnormal degradation rate of a variety of its components.

Cardiomyocyte hypertrophy, featuring contractile protein proliferation and other intracellular alterations, occurs in direct response to the abnormal loads of valvular diseases. Cardiomyocytes comprise a large proportion of the myocardium; therefore, hypertrophy of these cells necessarily results in overall cardiac, and particularly ventricular, hypertrophy. The nonmyocyte myocardial cellular elements (cardiac fibroblasts, endothelial cells, and some formed blood elements) also contribute to hypertrophy, however, by dividing and increasing in number, and by producing abnormal quantities of a variety of molecules that may be retained within the cell or may be secreted into the myocardial extracellular spaces. In the setting of valvular heart diseases, these remodeling processes can be understood in part as adaptive or compensatory responses to abnormal exogenous loading conditions to enable generation and transmission of contractile force sufficient for acceptable external work capacity and systemic homeostasis. In most instances, however, even if the changes are adaptive initially, they result in the deterioration of cardiac performance [4] when prolonged or particularly marked, eventually causing clinical sequelae.

Force generation versus force transmission

The function of the heart is to pump blood. This function requires active generation of contractile force. Consequently, the myocardial pathophysiology of valvular diseases must focus, at least in part, on the responses to exogenous loads of the contractile elements, organized in the sarcomere of the cardiomyocyte. Consistent with this focus, clinical prognostication in patients who have AR [5,6], AS [7], and MR [6,8] is closely related to contractility or to indices that reflect this intrinsic myocardial property.

Generation of force alone, however, is not sufficient to result in useful cardiac work. The force must be transmitted efficiently to other myocardial elements. Transmission must occur in a properly coordinated fashion along vectors that permit efficient contraction of the individual cardiomyocytes and of the myocardium as a whole. Thus, for example, generated force serves no useful purpose if it is simultaneously transmitted in diametrically opposite directions from the sarcomere. The pattern of force transmission is determined by a series of proteins that physically connect the sarcomere with the ECM [9]. Many of these proteins are produced by the cardiac fibroblast.

The importance of myocardial force transmission in supporting contractility has been highlighted during the past decade by observations in patients who have certain forms of muscular dystrophy [9–11] in which skeletal muscle weakness is associated with left ventricular systolic dysfunction and heart failure. Affected patients manifested point mutations resulting in deficient synthesis of dystrophins, proteins that serve as one of the direct links that physically connect the sarcomere to the ECM. In vitro, sarcomeres isolated from patients who have these forms of muscular dystrophy generate force normally. In vivo, however, force transmission is deficient and left ventricular performance is deranged. The deficiency of dystrophins is the basis of skeletal muscle and myocardial contractile deficiencies, leading to limb weakness and dilated cardiomyopathy/heart failure.

Though these studies were critical to the current understanding of force transmission and its importance, the dystrophins are only part of a series of "connector proteins" involved in force transmission. The force-generating sarcomere is linked to the dystrophins by elements of the actin cytoskeleton of the cardiomyocyte [9]. In turn, the dystrophins interact with the ECM via a glycoprotein complex located at the sarcolemma. This dystrophin-associated complex predominantly comprises fibronectin [9–13], a normal ECM component. If the actin cytoskeleton is deficient or structurally abnormal, if actin interactions with the dystrophins are defective, if dystrophins are deficient or qualitatively abnormal, if the glycoprotein complex is qualitatively or quantitatively abnormal, affecting its interaction with the dystrophins or with the ECM, or if abnormalities develop among integrins that may anchor links between the glycoprotein associated complex and elements of the ECM, force transmission must be affected. If force transmission is sufficiently deranged, heart failure may result. Thus, normal "myocyte-matrix interaction" must be reasonably preserved if contractility and cardiac mechanical function are to be sufficient to enable performance of life tasks within the envelope that is understood as "normal."

Recent research indicates that valvular diseases cause quantitative abnormalities in one or another of the ECM elements; the form and extent of these abnormalities depends on the specific exogenous overload (volume or pressure) and its magnitude. Though the precise mechanisms have not been fully elucidated, it appears quite likely that alterations of force transmission are important in defining the contractile response to valvular lesions. Concomitantly, variations in the ECM affect ventricular diastolic characteristics, potentially important contributors to the clinical response to valve diseases, discussed below.

Alterations in ECM components and connector proteins, as well as variations in the contractile elements, result largely from alterations in gene expression. These, in turn, cause a variety of quantitative alterations in signaling and enzyme pathways as well as in expression of specific structural peptides. When valve dysfunction is present, the alterations in gene expression are mediated by conditions that are peculiar to these diseases; such conditions include the abnormal mechanical stresses and strains that result directly from valvular stenosis or regurgitation. Transduction of these mechanical influences to gene (and protein) expression requires interaction of the stresses with the nuclear genetic material. Intracellular structural proteins are believed to mediate this interaction by transmitting mechanical stresses to the nucleus, which triggers variations in gene expression that result in the alterations in cellular synthetic and degradative processes [14],

defining the specific form of remodeling. Alternatively, it is possible that stresses induce alterations in signaling at the membrane level, perhaps by affecting ion channel activities or by changing configuration and hence, "activating" integrins and the like [15]. Indeed, "stress responsive" genomic elements have been described in the form of promoters that can be activated in response to specific mechanical stresses [16]; these provide a molecular explanation for this remodeling process.

Diastolic properties

The ECM is the "scaffold" on which the cardiomyocytes are organized. For this reason alone, the effects of stresses on fibroblast-mediated remodeling are intrinsically of interest. In addition, however, the characteristics of the ECM are primary determinants of the passive diastolic properties of the heart [4,17]. This function is subserved primarily by myocardial collagen, a structural protein with particular tensile strength. The specific quantitative characteristics of cardiac diastolic properties are modulated by the distribution of collagen isoforms: collagen type I, the predominant isoform in the normal heart, lacks crosslinks and allows normal compliance; collagen type III is cross-linked and reduces compliance. Any influence that increases the type III isoform in the left ventricle is likely to increase incremental ventricular diastolic pressure per increment in ventricular volume during diastolic filling. The result—abnormally high ventricular diastolic pressures at any ventricular volume—necessarily is reflected backward into the pulmonary vasculature to potentiate pulmonary vascular congestion and its resulting symptoms.

The luisotropic (active, oxygen-requiring relaxation) characteristics of the heart can result in diastolic phase abnormalities that alter chamber filling as well, and can lead to clinically important hemodynamic disturbances. The cardiomyocyte is responsible for active myocardial relaxation, as well as active contraction, and has some intrinsic elastic properties that affect other aspects of diastolic function.

Endothelial cells and leukocytes

Endothelial cells line the cardiac chambers and the myocardial vessels. Specific interactions between endothelial cells and myocardial remodeling have not been defined. Endothelial cells, however, can produce autocrine or paracrine factors in response to stress. These factors may affect local myocardial responses to environmental variations, though such factors remain to be explored. Leukocytes, which produce cytokines and other cell signaling molecules that modulate the molecular response to environmental variations [18], may be involved in the response to the overloads of valvular diseases, though these relations also have not yet been defined.

Cellular pathophysiology of valvular diseases

The cardiomyocyte

The response of the cardiomyocyte to pressure overload is hypertrophy [17,19]. When studied during the early days after initiation of the overload state, hypertrophy is largely driven by the abnormal synthesis of contractile proteins [20,21], particularly β-myosin heavy chain. Though the gross morphologic pattern of hypertrophy thereafter has led to the inference that continuing hypertrophy also is attributable to abnormal protein synthesis, little direct evidence has been developed to support this assumption.

Subcellular pathways transducing pressure loads to hypertrophy have been explored but are not understood completely. Modules of the mitogen-activated protein kinase (MAPK) cascade appear to be importantly involved [22]; from the authors' own work, at least one of these, the jun kinase (JNK) module, is involved in transducing the volume load of AR (as discussed later in the article), though the pattern of involvement appears to differ from that of pressure overload. In addition, several other factors have been implicated in the transduction of pressure overload, including specific G proteins, guanine triphosphatases, transforming growth factor β (TGF-β), fibroblast growth factor, insulin-like growth factor I receptor pathway, protein kinase C, calcineurin, and others [22]. In vitro experiments suggest that whereas the hypertrophied cardiomyocyte of left ventricular pressure overload maintains grossly normal functional characteristics, subtle evidence of contractile dysfunction may be present from an early time, perhaps due to abnormal expression of the β-myosin heavy chain [20]. Experimental data have been supplemented by observations from studies of myocardial biopsies obtained in humans during valve surgery. These data have provided evidence that, by the time of surgery for AS, autophagy, oncosis, and apoptosis affect cardiomyocytes [4]; these processes are likely to diminish the cardiomyocyte cell number when

compared with normal and with earlier stages of the natural history of the disease.

Experimental evidence also suggests that cardiomyocyte connexins, the proteins that comprise gap junctions, are down-regulated by AS [23,24]. Connexins are believed to be centrally involved in the intercellular transmission of electrical signals at the intercalated discs; hypothetically, their alteration may create the substrate for clinically important cardiac arrhythmias.

Alterations in energy metabolism have been suggested experimentally. The pattern of substrate use differs between physiologic and pathologic cardiac hypertrophy, such that in physiologic hypertrophy there is increased use of long-chain fatty acids and decreased use of glucose, whereas in pathologic conditions, the reverse occurs [25]. These differences in energy use may affect gene expression and cardiac remodeling via oxidative mechanisms [26].

The cardiomyocyte response in volume overload is importantly different from the pattern associated with pressure overload. Moreover, the pathophysiology of the cardiomyocyte differs in volume loading caused by AR compared with volume loading caused by MR. These differences probably are rooted in the dissimilarities of the mechanical alterations caused by the two lesions. AR imposes abnormal wall stresses/afterload on the left ventricle from the moment the lesion is initiated; in contrast, MR is characterized by rapid left ventricular emptying, enabled by availability of the low impedance retrograde left atrial egress pathway, with consequent maintenance of normal left ventricular wall stresses/afterload until other factors cause myocyte functional deterioration.

As in AS, cellular hypertrophy occurs in AR (though characterized by a morphologically different pattern than in AS [19]) and features abnormal contractile protein content. However, within several days after the initiation of experimental AR, the metabolic basis underlying increasing intracellular content of contractile proteins is not abnormal synthesis but rather subnormal contractile protein degradation [27–29]. The functional consequences of the accumulation of "old" contractile proteins are not clear yet, and the complex signaling pathways leading to this development remain to be elucidated. Similarly, suppression of myocardial protein degradation also appears to underlie the less marked left ventricular hypertrophy associated with MR [30]. More importantly, however, cardiomyocyte dysfunction in

MR appears to be associated with variations in sympathetic nervous system activity [31], characterized by abnormal rates of norepinephrine secretion (and reuptake) by myocardial sympathetic nerve terminals. These abnormalities occur before evidence of contractile dysfunction, and increase as disordered contractility and clinical debility supervene; these findings appear to reflect the known toxic effects of sustained norepinephrine application on cardiomyocytes, including stimulation of proinflammatory cytokine production [32], and ultimately leading to apoptosis.

Finally, as opposed to the upregulation of connexins found in the pressure overload of AS, down-regulation, at least of connexin 43, is associated with the mechanical strains of AR [33]. As for AS, this abnormality in AR ultimately may predispose to clinically important arrhythmia, though a specific relation remains to be elucidated.

The cardiac fibroblast and the extracellular matrix

Myocardial fibrosis is the net result of synthesis and degradation of the various ECM elements, which include collagen, glycoproteins, proteoglycans, glycosoaminoglycans, and fibroblasts. ECM synthesis depends upon the transcription and translation of genes coding for specific ECM components. This activity is primarily, or solely, the function of the cardiac fibroblast, though some experimental data suggests that a somewhat dedifferentiated "myofibroblast" often is the responsible cell [34]. ECM degradation depends upon the relative activity of matrix metaloproteases (MMPs) that cleave and degrade peptides [35], and endogenous tissue inhibitors of metaloproteases (TIMPs) [36], also primarily produced by the fibroblast. The MMP/TIMP system can decrease the fibrous tissue content of the myocardium or remodel the ECM by altering the proportions of specific components.

When the left ventricle is pathologically pressure loaded, as in AS or systemic hypertension, available evidence indicates that the marked fibrotic response [4,17,19,37] is characterized by a noticeable increase in collagen content compared with normal collagen content, caused by enhanced gene expression and protein synthesis [38,39]. Though fibronectin content also may be abnormal [4], the magnitude of this change probably is disproportionately less than that of collagen.

MMPs for collagen isoforms 1, 2, and 3 are increased modestly, but TIMPs 1 and 2 are increased to a disproportionately greater extent [40,41]. These may not be all the MMPs and TIMPs involved in collagen metabolism; however, this pattern for these measurable enzymes suggests that though collagen turnover is increased as indicated by the abnormal MMP activity, remodeling–degradation is modest compared with synthesis. Myocardial collagen content increases, therefore, with synthesis greater than degradation.

These ECM changes contribute to the maintenance of normal left ventricular chamber size and subnormal left ventricular compliance. Lack of ventricular dilatation, coupled with ventricular wall thickening (concentric hypertrophy), helps to minimize afterload excess caused by the pressure overload, though the loss of compliance undoubtedly contributes to symptom development.

The volume overload of AR causes a dramatically different myocardial response. Experimental evidence indicates that collagen content is normal initially despite abnormal wall stresses and strains, and tends to fall to subnormal by the time heart failure develops [42]. In an experimental model of AR, genes coding for collagen isoforms are expressed normally, indicating a lack of significantly abnormal or subnormal synthetic activity (preliminary data from human biopsies at surgery, now being analyzed in the authors' laboratory, suggest a similar pattern in humans) [13,43,44]. In preliminary results obtained in fibroblast cell cultures from animals with surgically induced AR, however, activity of MMPs 1 and 2 is almost three times normal, while activity of TIMPs is modestly but significantly subnormal [45]. This pattern of enzyme expression may contribute to the absence of collagen content abnormalities, even in severe AR with heart failure. Though total collagen content is little affected by the volume load of AR, however, collagen isoform proportions are abnormal [46]; from the authors' preliminary data, type II collagen (cross-linked, providing high tensile strength and tending to minimize ventricular compliance) is represented disproportionately in the myocardium. This finding may be explained by the capacity of specific MMPs to cleave specific isoforms, altering their proportional distribution and resulting in remodeling of ECM components like collagen and, hence, of the ECM itself, without altering net ECM content.

It may be inferred that because collagen content fails to increase, the left ventricle in AR is not structurally adapted to resist volume loading, but that its structure permits continuing dilatation with the development of increasing wall stresses. This sequence of events, a so-called "vicious cycle," tends to perpetuate remodeling of the ECM and the contractile protein metabolic alterations in cardiomyocytes previously described. Though hypothetical, this pathophysiology is consistent with the observed alterations and provides a plausible basis for the clinical observation that "regurgitation begets regurgitation."

At first glance, stability of myocardial collagen content would seem to be discordant with the observation that fibrosis is prominent in the left ventricles of animals with experimental AR [47] as well as in humans with this disease [48]. However, whereas myocardial collagen content is unchanged by AR, glycoprotein content is doubled or tripled. Cell cultures of fibroblasts isolated from the myocardium of rabbits with surgically induced chronic AR and from the myocardium of normal rabbits exhibit markedly abnormal expression of genes coding for fibronectin [13,44,49]. Thrombospondin, another glycoprotein, is similarly overexpressed in AR, while amyloid prescursor protein expression is twice normal. These results have been confirmed in experiments in which normal cardiac fibroblasts are exposed in culture to physical strains that model those found at the left ventricular midwall in severe AR [13,44,50].

Moreover, the AR-induced abnormalities of gene expression are translated into parallel abnormalities in protein expression. Thus, glucosamine, a substrate for fibronectin and other glycoproteins, is taken up markedly abnormally and avidly by AR (or strained) fibroblasts (Fig. 1) [44], and Western analyses of the products of cultured fibroblasts (normal versus AR, and strained versus nonstrained normal cells) indicate that AR induces abnormal expression of fibronectin, the magnitude of which is directly related to the magnitude of AR [44]. Because fibronectin appears to be importantly involved in the physical interaction of myocyte and matrix that underlies normal force transmission, alteration of ECM fibronectin content may derange force transmission, compromising contractility and contributing to ventricular dysfunction and heart failure.

Identification of tissue collagen/fibronectin distribution and proportions—with appropriately tagged tracers or other imaging approaches, or with quantitation of metabolites released into blood—may add importantly to current methods for prognostication. Additionally, molecular or pharmacologic blockade of gene expression or translation, if properly targeted specifically to myocardial tissue and with an acceptably safe ratio of therapeutic to toxic activity, could forestall the development of pathologic fibrosis and thus enhance collagen-mediated resistance to left ventricular dilatation while limiting impediments to normal force transmission.

Such prognostic and therapeutic developments require a considerable amount of additional research, including the definition of the cellular and molecular pathways by which mechanical stresses and strains are transduced to alterations in gene

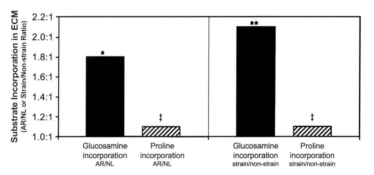

Fig. 1. Glucosamine or proline incorporated into extracellular matrix by cardiac fibroblasts (CF), illustrating relatively enhanced uptake and use of the substrate for glycoproteins, but not for collagen, by CF in AR compared with normal. (*Left*) Incorporation by CF from AR hearts, expressed as a ratio normalized to incorporation by normal CF. (*Right*) Incorporation by normal CF cultured during exogenous mechanical strain, expressed as a ratio normalized to incorporation by normal CF cultured without mechanical strain. *$P = .001$, glucosamine incorporation by AR CF versus paired normal CF. **$P < .001$, glucosamine incorporation by strained normal CF versus paired normal nonstrained CF. †Not significant, proline incorporation by AR CF versus paired normal CF and strained normal CF versus nonstrained CF. (*From* Borer JS, Truter SL, Herrold EM, et al. Myocardial fibrosis in chronic aortic regurgitation: molecular and cellular response to volume overload. Circulation 2002;105:1839; with permission.)

and protein expression. Recent preliminary experimental data in the authors' laboratory indicate that the mechanical strain of AR results in alteration of the proportions of specific subunits comprising fibroblast integrins that serve as binding sites for ECM proteins (the perturbation of these integrins also is involved in fibronectin synthesis); these findings are consistent with earlier demonstrations that mechanical factors can modulate integrin expression [14]. Parallel studies in our laboratory indicate that the mechanical strain of AR specifically stimulates the JNK module of the intracytoplasmic MAPK cascade. JNK activation stimulates cyclic adenosine monophosphate-response element located in the fibronectin gene promoter [51,52]. Preliminarily, JNK stimulation also enhances activity of MMPs 1 and 2, tending to suppress myocardial collagen content in AR, as has been reported in other systems [53]. Thus, both suppression of normal collagen metabolism (potentially precluding resistance to pathologic left ventricular dilatation) and promotion of abnormal fibronectin production (potentially deranging force transmission) are mediated in part by the JNK module in the cardiac fibroblast.

Additional data must be developed before the configuration of practical pharmacologic approaches to normalization of ECM metabolism. Experimental and clinical pharmacologic data, however, suggest the relevance of these observations for current therapy.

Implications for conventional drug therapy

In theory, any drug that reduces impedance to left ventricular outflow is beneficial in AR and MR by counteracting the mechanical forces that drive regurgitant blood flow. This has led to the suggestion that vasodilating drugs, and particularly angiotensin-converting enzyme inhibitors (of great value in the treatment of patients who have heart failure of nonvalvular causes), may be employed in patients with AR and MR to forestall myocardial dysfunction [54]. This strategy is appropriate, however, only if (1) clinically and prognostically useful myocardial salvage can be affected by the extent of impedance lowering achievable clinically with these agents; and (2) other actions of the drugs employed, in addition to vasodilatation (all drugs have multiple pharmacologic effects), do not result in clinical harm that outweighs the putative benefit of vasodilatation. Studies after short-duration vasodilator

administration [55,56] and after several months of drug administration [57–60] have demonstrated drug-mediated improvement in ventricular performance. However, recent studies involving a longer duration of drug use, extending through several years, suggest important differences in clinical responses. Thus, in randmonized prospective trials, long-acting nifedipine, administered to predominantly hypertensive patients with AR, seems clearly to forestall development of heart failure and of left ventricular functional deterioration that warrants surgery in asymptomatic patients [61,62]; more recent data from a prospectively designed randomized trial in a population characterized by near normal blood pressure [63] showed no benefit from this strategy. Conversely, the latter study suggests that an angiotensin-converting enzyme inhibitor in such patients may be detrimental, a conclusion that is supported by a retrospective analysis of a large, prospectively designed epidemiologic study from the authors' program [64]. In MR, very few relevant data exist. In the only prospective trial focusing on the clinical outcome of drug therapy for nonischemic MR, however, recent data indicate that an angiotensin-converting enzyme inhibitor was associated with significant clinical deterioration, in comparison with a placebo, in patients treated for 1year [65], a finding that is anticipated by several experimental studies that suggest the potential detriment of blockade of the renin–angiotensin system in MR [66–69].

The basis for these findings may reside in the effects of these drugs on the ECM. Thus, dihydropyridine calcium channel blocking drugs like nifedipine are not known to affect the ECM in any substantial manner, whereas angiotensin blockade, either by converting enzyme inhibitors or receptor blockers, block collagen synthesis [70] (probably by impeding TGF-β activity) and thus potentially preclude development of necessary structural support of the left ventricle to resist dilatation. While this explanation is hypothetical and must be tested by appropriately designed studies, emerging knowledge of the pathobiology of valvular diseases and empirical data from the clinical trials described in this section suggest that, at the very least, it is necessary to rethink the role of vasodilator therapy for regurgitant valvular diseases. These data suggest that if any drug therapy is to be useful, it must be directed at cellular/molecular processes importantly involved in the pathophysiology of myocardial functional deterioration and not on nonspecific vasodilatation.

Summary

Much remains to be learned about the patho-biology of valvular heart diseases at the cellular and molecular levels. It seems clear at this point, however, that important pathophysiologic differences exist between the responses to left ventricular pressure loading (AS) and to volume loading (AR and MR), and similarly important differences exist in the responses to the two volume-loading lesions, based on the dissimilarities in mechanical stresses and strains that impact on the left ventricle from these lesions. The effects of these mechanical influences are felt by myocardial cardiomyocytes and fibroblasts, and perhaps by other cellular elements. The pathophysiology of myocardial dysfunction is undoubtedly the net result of metabolic alterations and remodeling of the structure and secretory activities of these different cell lines. As increasing knowledge further elucidates the mechanisms by which abnormal mechanical influences are transduced to disordered myocardial cell biology, it is reasonable to foresee a time when the clinical debility associated with valve diseases will be mitigated by nonsurgical modulation of myocardial biology and the decision to apply direct mechanical therapy will be undertaken based on interrogation of cellular processes with precision that is not currently possible.

References

[1] Borer JS, Schuleri K. Myocardial remodeling: physiological and pathological. In: Greenberg B, editor. Myocardial remodeling: mechanisms and treatment. New York: Taylor and Francis; 2006. p. 121–38.

[2] Leri A, Kajstura J, Anversa P. Cardiac stem cells and mechanisms of myocardial regeneration. Physiol Rev 2005;85:1373–416.

[3] Sonnenblick EH, Anversa P. Models and remodeling: mechanisms and clinical implications. Cardiologia 1999;44:609–19.

[4] Hein S, Arnon E, Kostin S, et al. Progression from compensated hypertrophy to failure in the pressure-overloaded human heart: structural deterioration and compensatory mechanisms. Circulation 2003;107:984–91.

[5] Borer JS, Hochreiter C, Herrold EM, et al. Prediction of indications for valve replacement among asymptomatic or minimally symptomatic patients with chronic aortic regurgitation and normal left ventricular performance. Circulation 1998;97:525–34.

[6] Borer JS, Bonow RO. Contemporary approach to aortic and mitral regurgitation. Circulation 2003;108:2432–8.

[7] de Filippi CR, Willett DL, Brickner ME, et al. Usefulness of dobutamine echocardiography in distinguishing severe from nonsevere valvular aortic stenosis in patients with depressed left ventricular function and low transvalvular gradients. Am J Cardiol 1995;75:191–4.

[8] Sarano ME, Tajik AJ, Schaff HV, et al. Echocardiographic prediction of survival after surgical correction of organic mitral regurgitation. Circulation 1994;90:830–7.

[9] Leiden J. The genetics of dilated cardiomyopathy: emerging clues to the puzzle. N Engl J Med 1997;337:1080–1.

[10] Towbin JA. Role of cytoskeletal proteins in cardiomyopathies. Current Opinions in Cell Biology 1998;10:131–9.

[11] Bowles NE, Bowles KR, Towbin JA. The "final common pathway" hypothesis and inherited cardiovascular disease: the role of cytoskeletal proteins in dilated cardiomyopathy. Herz 2000;25:168–75.

[12] Ahumada G, Saffitz J. Fibronectin in the rat heart: link between cardiac myocytes and collagen. J Histochem Cytochem 1984;32:383–8.

[13] Borer JS, Truter SL, Herrold EM, et al. The cellular and molecular basis of heart failure in regurgitant valvular diseases: the myocardial extracellular matrix as a building block for future therapy. Adv Cardiol 2002;39:7–14.

[14] MacKenna D, Dolfi F, Vuori K, et al. Extracellular signal-regulated kinase and c-Jun NH2-terminal kinase activation by mechanical stretch is integrin-dependant and matrix-specific in rat cardiac fibroblasts. J Clin Invest 1998;101:301–10.

[15] Ravens U. Mechano-electric feedback and arrhythmias. Prog Biophys Mol Biol 2003;82:255–66.

[16] Gimbroni M, Najel T, Topper J. Biochemical activation: an emerging paradigm in endothelial adhesion biology. J Clin Invest 1997;99:1809–13.

[17] Hess OM, Schneider J, Koch R, et al. Diastolic function and myocardial structure in patients with myocardial hypertrophy. Circulation 1981;63:360–71.

[18] Weihrauch D, Arras M, Zimmermann R, et al. Importance of monocytes/macrophages and fibroblasts for healing of micronecroses in porcine myocardium. Mol Cell Biochem 1995;147:13–9.

[19] Maron BJ, Ferrans VJ, Roberts WC. Myocardial ultrastructure in patients with chronic aortic valve disease. Am J Cardiol 1975;35:725–31.

[20] Dorn GW, Robbins J, Ball N, et al. Myosin heavy chain regulation and myocyte contractile depression after LV hypertrophy in aortic-banded mice. Am J Physiol 1994;267:H400–5.

[21] Nagai R, Pritzl N, Low RB, et al. Myosin isozyme synthesis and mRNA levels in pressure overloaded rabbit hearts. Circ Res 1987;60:692–9.

[22] Molkentin JD, Dorn GW. Cytoplasmic signaling pathways that regulate cardiac hypertrophy. Annu Rev Physiol 2001;63:391–426.

[23] Peters NS, Green CR, Poole-Wilson PA, et al. Reduced content of connexin43 gap junctions in ventricular myocardium from hypertrophied and ischemic human hearts. Circulation 1993;88: 864–75.

[24] Peters N. New insights into myocardial arrhythmogenesis: distribution of gap-junctional coupling in normal, ischaemic and hypertrophied human hearts. Clin Sci 1996;90:447–52.

[25] Allard MF. Energy substrate metabolism in cardiac hypertrophy. Curr Hypertens Rep 2004;6: 430–5.

[26] Ungvari Z, Gupte SA, Recchia FA, et al. Role of oxidative-nitrosative stress and downstream pathways in various forms of cardiomyopathy and heart failure. Curr Vasc Pharmacol 2005;3:221–9.

[27] Magid NM, Borer JS, Young MS, et al. Suppression of protein degradation in progressive cardiac hypertrophy of chronic aortic regurgitation. Circulation 1993;87:1249–57.

[28] Magid NM, Wallerson DC, Borer JS. Myofibrillar protein turnover in cardiac hypertrophy due to aortic regurgitation. Cardiology 1993;82:20–9.

29 King RK, Magid NM, Opio G, et al. Protein turnover in compensated chronic aortic regurgitation. Cardiology 1997;88:518–25.

[30] Matsuo T, Carabello BA, Nagatomo Y, et al. Mechanisms of cardiac hypertrophy in canine volume overload. Am J Physiol 1998;275(Pt 2):H65–74.

[31] Starling MR. Emerging biology of mitral regurgitation: implications for further therapy. Adv Cardiol 2002;39:15–24.

[32] Murray DF, Prabhu SD, Chandrasekar B. Chronic β adrenergic stimulation induces myocardial proinflammatory cytokine expression. Circulation 2000; 101:2338–41.

[33] Goldfine SM, Walcott B, Brink PR, et al. Myocardial connexin43 expression in left ventricular hypertrophy resulting from aortic regurgitation. Cardiovasc Pathol 1999;8:1–6.

[34] Eghbali M, Tomek R, Woods C, et al. Cardiac fibroblasts are predisposed to convert into myocyte phenotype: specific effect of TGFb. Proc Natl Acad Sci USA 1991;88:795–9.

[35] Tyagi SC, Lewis K, Pikes D, et al. Stretch-induced membrane type matrix metalloproteinase and tissue plasminogen activator in cardiac fibroblast cells. J Cell Physiol 1998;176:374–82.

[36] Woessner JF Jr. Matrix metalloproteinases and their inhibitors in connective tissue remodeling. FASEB J 1991;5:2145–54.

[37] Schwarz F, Flaming W, Schaper J, et al. Myocardial structure and function in patients with aortic valve disease and their relation to post-operative results. Am J Cardiol 1978;441:661–8.

[38] Weber KT, Janicki JS, Shroff SG, et al. Collagen remodeling of the pressure overloaded, hypertrophied non-human primate myocardium. Circ Res 1988;62:757–65.

[39] Weber KT, Brilla CG. Pathological hypertrophy and the cardiac interstitium. Circulation 1991;83: 1849–65.

[40] Janicki JS, Brower GL, Gardner JD, et al. The dynamic interaction between matrix metalloproteinase activity and adverse myocardial remodeling. Heart Fail Rev 2004;9:33–42.

[41] Tayebjee MH, MacFadyen RJ, Lip GY. Extracellular matrix biology: a new frontier in linking the pathology and therapy of hypertension? J Hypertens 2003;21:2211–8.

[42] Goldfine SM, Pena M, Magid NM, et al. Myocardial collagen in cardiac hypertrophy resulting from chronic aortic regurgitation. Am J Ther 1998;5: 139–46.

[43] Truter SL, Goldin D, Kolesar J, et al. Abnormal gene expression of cardiac fibroblasts in experimental aortic regurgitation. Am J Ther 2000;7:237–43.

[44] Borer JS, Truter SL, Herrold EM, et al. Myocardial fibrosis in chronic aortic regurgitation: molecular and cellular response to volume overload. Circulation 2002;105:1837–42.

[45] Schuleri K, Lee E, Pitlor LL, Truter SL, et al. Subnormal tissue inhibitor of metalloproteinase expression modulates matrix metalloproteinase-2 activity and fibrosis in aortic regurgitation. J Am Coll Cardiol 2004;43:A431–2.

[46] Piper C, Schultheiss HP, Akdemir D, et al. Remodeling of the cardiac extracellular matrix differs between volume- and pressure-overloaded ventricles and is specific for each heart valve lesion. J Heart Valve Dis 2003;12:592–600.

[47] Liu SK, Magid NM, Fox PR, et. Fibrosis, myocyte degeneration and heart failure in chronic experimental aortic regurgitation. Cardiology 1998;90: 101–9.

[48] Krayenbuhl HP, Hess OM, Monrad ES, et al. Left ventricular mnyocardial structure in aortic valve disease before, intermediate and late after aortic valve replacement. Circulation 1989;79:744–55.

[49] Borer JS, Truter SL, Gupta A, et al. Heart failure in aortic regurgitation: the role of primary fibrosis and its cellular and molecular pathophysiology. Adv Cardiol 2004;41:16–24.

[50] Gupta A, Carter J, Truter SL, et al. Cellular response of human cardiac fibroblasts to mechanically simulated aortic regurgitation. Am J Ther 2006;13: 8–11.

[51] Truter SL, Dumlao TF, Lee E, et al. Over-expression of fibronectin involves activation of mitogen-activated protein-kinase-kinase of the stress activated protein kinase/C-Jun N-terminal kinase in aortic regulation. J Am Coll Cardiol 2004; 43:A430–1.

[52] Truter SL, Gupta A, Leer EH, et al. The stress-activated protein kinase pathways, C-jun N-terminal kinase and P38 mitogen activated protein kinase, regulate fibronectin expression in aortic regurgitation. J Am Coll Cardiol 2005;45:353A.

[53] Li YS, Shyy JY, Li S, Lee J, et al. The Ras-JNK pathway is involved in shear-induced gene expression. Mol Cell Biol 1996;16:5947–54.

[54] Bonow RO, Carabello BA, Chatterjee K, et al. ACC/AHA 2006 guidelines for the management of patients with valvular heart disease—executive summary: a report of the American College of Cardiology/American Heart Association Task Force on Practice Guidelines (Writing Committee to Revise the 1998 Guidelines for the Management of Patients with Valvular Heart Disease). J Am Coll Cardiol 2006;48:598–675.

[55] Borer JS, Bonow RO, Bacharach SL, et al. The effects of nitroglycerin in patients with valvular heart disease: hemodynamic and radionuclide cineangiographic studies. In: Litchtlen PR, Engel HJ, editors. Proceedings of the Third International Symposium on Nitrates, Monte Carlo, 1980. Berlin: Springer-Verlag; 1981. p. 546–51.

[56] Borer JS, Redwood DR, Itscoitz SB, et al. Nitroglycerin-induced improvement in exercise tolerance and hemodynamics in patients with chronic rheumatic valvular heart disease. Am J Cardiol 1978;41:302–7.

[57] Greenberg B, Massie B, Bristow JD, et al. Long-term vasodilator therapy of chronic aortic insufficiency: a randomized double-blinded placebo-controlled clinical trial. Circulation 1988;78:92–103.

[58] Scognamiglio R, Fasoli G, Ponchia A, et al. Long-term nifedipine unloading therapy in asymptomatic patients with chronic severe aortic regurgitation. J Am Coll Cardiol 1990;16:424–9.

[59] Jensen T, Kornerup J, Lederballe O, et al. Treatment with hydralazine in mild to moderate mitral or aortic incompetence. Eur Heart J 1983;4:306–12.

[60] Wisenbaugh T, Sinovich V, Dullabh A, et al. Six month pilot study of captopril for mildly symptomatic, severe isolated mitral and isolated aortic regurgitation. J Heart Valve Dis 1994;3:197–204.

[61] Scognamiglio R, Rahimtoola SH, Fasoli G, et al. Nifedipine in asymptomatic patients with severe aortic regurgitation and normal left ventricular function. N Engl J Med 1994;331:689–94.

[62] Scognamiglio R, Negut C, Palisi M, et al. Long-term survival and functional results after aortic valve replacement in asymptomatic patients with chronic severe aortic regurgitation and left ventricular dysfunction. J Am Coll Cardiol 2005;45:1025–30.

[63] Evangelista A, Tornos P, Sambola A, et al. Long-term vasodilator therapy in patients with severe aortic regurgitation. N Engl J Med 2005;353:1342–9.

[64] Supino PG, Borer JS, Prebisz J, et al. Prognostic impact of systolic hypertension on asymptomatic patients with chronic severe aortic regurgitation and initially normal left ventricular performance at rest. Am J Cardiol 2005;96:964–70.

[65] Sampaio RO, Grinberg M, Leite JJ, et al. Effect of enalapril on left ventricular diameters and exercise capacity in asymptomatic or mildly symptomatic patients with regurgitation secondary to mitral valve prolapse or rheumatic heart disease. Am J Cardiol 2005;96:117–21.

[66] Nemoto S, Masayoshi Hamawaki M, Gilberto De Freitas G, et al. Differential effects of the angiotensin-converting enzyme inhibitor lisinopril versus the beta-adrenergic receptor blocker atenolol on hemodynamics and left ventricular contractile function in experimental mitral regurgitation. J Am Coll Cardiol 2002;40:149–54.

[67] Dell'Italia LJ, Balcells E, Meng QC, et al. Volume-overload cardiac hypertrophy is unaffected by ACE inhibitor treatment in dogs. Am J Physiol 1997;273(2 Pt 2):H961–70.

[68] Perry GJ, Wei CC, Hankes GH, et al. Angiotensin II receptor blockade does not improve left ventricular function and remodeling in subacute mitral regurgitation in the dog. J Am Coll Cardiol 2002;39:1374–9.

[69] Dell'Italia LJ, Meng QC, Balcells E, et al. Increased ACE and chymase-like activity in cardiac tissue of dogs with chronic mitral regurgitation. Am J Physiol 1995;269:H2065–73.

[70] Brilla CG, Zhou G, Matsubara L, et al. Collagen metabolism in cultured adult rat cardiac fibroblasts: response to angiotensin II and aldosterone. J Mol Cell Cardiol 1994;26:809–20.

ELSEVIER
SAUNDERS

Heart Failure Clin 2 (2006) 425–433

HEART
FAILURE
CLINICS

Assessment of Mitral Regurgitation and Clinical Decision-Making

Geu-Ru Hong, MD, Peng Li, MD, PhD, Walter Tsang, MD,
Mani A. Vannan, MBBS, FACC*

University of California Irvine, Orange, CA, USA

Echocardiography is key to the assessment of both the etiology and severity of regurgitation (Table 1). It also provides important clinical information regarding left ventricular size and function, left atrial size, and pulmonary arterial pressure. Doppler detection of valve regurgitation has been a standard clinical tool for more than 20 years. Color and spectral Doppler echocardiography still serves as a screening tool and quantifies mitral regurgitation (MR) with vena contracta, which is used to identify patients who require further evaluation. The quantitation of valve regurgitation parameters broadly includes the calculation of the volume of backflow across the valve (regurgitant volume[RV]), the percent regurgitation as compared with the total stroke volume (regurgitant fraction [RF]), and the effective regurgitant orifice (ERO) area. Though the RV and RF depend on the driving pressure across the valve and the ERO may vary with valve dynamics, all of these measures are more accurate and reproducible than older parameters, such as the regurgitant jet length or area on Doppler echocardiography [1–4].

Assessment of feasibility and results of repair

Echocardiography is important in selecting patients with MR in whom valve repair is feasible. Mitral valve disease caused by rheumatic valvular disease or endocarditis is more difficult to repair

and is more likely to be treated with valve replacement [5]. Echocardiography is useful not only in predicting the feasibility of valve repair, but also in the assessment of the adequacy of the valve repair at the time of surgery. Intraoperative transesophageal echocardiography (TEE) is performed routinely to assess the adequacy of mitral valve repair by detecting any residual stenosis or regurgitation [6]. When satisfactory repair cannot be achieved, replacement of the valve at the time of the mitral valve operation is preferred over performing the valve replacement operation at a later date.

Semiquantitative assessment of mitral regurgitation

Semiquantitative methods of assessing MR include continuous wave (CW) Doppler echocardiography, Doppler color flow imaging, measurement of vena contracta [7–9], and assessment of pulmonary venous velocity [10].

Continuous wave Doppler

The severity of MR can be assessed semiquantitatively using CW Doppler echocardiography. The intensity of the MR signal depends upon the intensity of the transmitted wave, as well as the attenuation of the reflected wave (a function of depth) and the number of erythrocytes [11]. Thus, a spectral Doppler of MR—which is as dense as the spectral envelope of the antegrade mitral flow—indicates severe MR. This may be unreliable when the interrogating Doppler sample volume is not adequately aligned with the

* Corresponding author. University of California Irvine, 101 The City Drive, Building 53, Route 81, Orange, CA 92868-4080.

  E-mail address: mvannan@uci.edu (M.A. Vannan).

1551-7136/06/$ - see front matter © 2007 Elsevier Inc. All rights reserved.
doi:10.1016/j.hfc.2007.02.002

Table 1
Role of echocardiography in mitral regurgitation

Morphologic assessment of the mitral valve
- Assessment of feasibility of repair of mitral regurgitation

Assessment of the degree of mitral regurgitation
- Semi-quantitative methods
  Continuous wave Doppler
  Color Doppler flow imaging
  Pulmonary venous velocities
- Quantitative methods
  Vena contracta (VC) width
  Effective regurgitant orifice (ERO)
  Regurgitant volume (RV)
  Regurgitant fraction (RF)

Assessment of consequences of mitral regurgitation
- Assessment of left ventricular function
- Assessment of left atrial size

regurgitant jet. The contour of the spectral envelope of the MR jet also indicates the severity of MR in the patient. In patients with acute or subacute severe MR, early systolic peaking of the MR velocity by a continuous wave occurs, reflecting an early rise in left atrial pressure [11]. However, the effect of severe MR on ventricular size and function is determined not only by the

severity of the regurgitation but also by the duration of the regurgitation. Severe MR that occurs in the latter half of systole is seen frequently, and may occur with relatively modest effects on ventricular and atrial size; thus, it may be of less risk in causing contractile dysfunction [12].

Color Doppler flow imaging

Color Doppler flow imaging provides a method for the detection of the direction and extent of the regurgitant jet in the left atrium. Jet length, jet to left atrial area ratio, and more simply, jet area [13] have been used as indices of MR severity (Table 2). Although the extent of MR by color Doppler flow imaging allows the severity of the patient's MR to be assessed rapidly, this imaging method may not always be accurate. Many technical factors, including sector size, color gain, and Nyquist limit, can affect the size of the regurgitant jet independently of the regurgitant orifice [14].

Pulmonary venous velocities

Pulmonary venous velocity profile is useful in assessing the degree of MR [10]. Systolic reversal in pulmonary veins is strong evidence for severe MR; it is not only related to the severity of MR,

Table 2
Qualitative and quantitative parameters useful in grading mitral regurgitation severity

	Mild	Moderate		Severe
Structural parameters				
LA size	Normal	Normal or dilated		Usually dilated
LV size	Normal	Normal or dilated		Usually dilated
Doppler parameters				
Color flow jet area	Small central jet (<4 cm^2 or $<20\%$ of LA area)	Variable		Large central jet (>10 cm^2 or $>40\%$ of LA area)
Mitral inflow (PW)	A wave dominant	Variable		E-wave dominant
Jet density (CW)	Incomplete or faint	Dense		Dense
Jet contour (CW)	Parabolic	Usually parabolic		Early peaking-triangular
Pulmonary vein flow	Systolic dominance	Systolic blunting		Systolic flow reversal
Quantitative parameters				
VC width (cm)	<0.3	0.3–0.69		≥ 0.7
R Vol (ml/beat)	<30	30–44	45–59	≥ 60
RF (%)	<30	30–39	40–49	≥ 50
ERO (cm^2)	<0.2	0.20–0.29	0.30–0.39	≥ 0.40

Abbreviations: LA, left atrium; LV, left ventricle; PW, pulsed wave; R Vol, regurgitant volume; VC, vena contracta.
Modified from Zoghbi WA, Enriquez-Sarano M, Faster B, et al. Recommendations for evaluation of the severity of native valvular regurgitation with two dimensional and Doppler echocardiography. J Am Soc Echocardiogr 2003;16:777–802.

but also to jet direction and left atrial pressure. Conversely, pulmonary venous reversal may be absent or asymmetric in patients who have severe MR. Systolic pulmonary venous blunting and reversal, both useful signs of severe MR, have relatively low sensititivity [15].

Quantitative assessment of mitral regurgitation

Quantitative methods include assessment of RV, RF, and ERO based on the continuity equation and the proximal isovelocity surface area methods [16–18], and direct measurement of vena contracta as an index of ERO (see Table 2). MR is classified as severe when the ERO is 0.40 mm², the regurgitant fraction is 50%, the regurgitant volume is 60 mL/beat [19], or VC diameter is >0.7 mm.

Vena contracta

The vena contracta is the region of regurgitant flow immediately below the flow convergence through the regurgitant orifice [20]. The width of the vena contracta has been demonstrated to increase directly in relation to the size of the regurgitant orifice. This relationship exists relatively independently of driving pressure and flow rate in clinical ranges [9]. Therefore, direct measurement of the vena contracta width provides an index of ERO. The vena contracta width seems superior to jet measurements and can be obtained by either TEE [20] or transthoracic echocardiography [7,8]. Standard transthoracic windows can measure jet height (parasternal long axis) and crosssectional area (parasternal short axis). A jet height of 0.5 cm indicates moderate to severe MR, whereas a width of 0.3 cm indicates mild MR (Fig. 1) [4].

Two dimensional echo and Doppler approaches

One way to calculate RV and RF is to estimate the mitral and aortic stroke volumes using pulsed wave Doppler echocardiography [16]. The principle is simple and applicable in most cases, but the measurement of the mitral stroke volume is technically demanding, with a significant learning curve [16]. In patients who have MR, the total stroke volume is equal to the systemic stroke volume plus the RV. The systemic stroke volume is usually calculated at the left ventricle outflow tract (LVOT), provided that there is no significant aortic regurgitation.

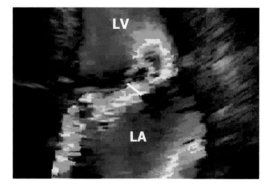

Fig. 1. Color flow recording of a MR jet—a zoomed view in the apical view. Color Doppler showing severe mitral insufficiency caused by posterior leaflet prolapse. The severity of insufficiency is directly related to the width of the vena contracta of the jet. LA, left atrium; LV, left ventricle. (*From* Vannan MA, Liu Z, Rakowski H, et al, editors. Atlas of heart diseases: echocardiography. Philadelphia: Current Medicine LLC; 2005. © 2005, Current Medicine LLC; used with permission.)

It is the product of the cross-sectional area (CSA) and the time velocity integral (TVI) at the LVOT. The total stroke volume is the stroke volume that passes through the mitral valve. This is the product of the CSA and the TVI at the mitral annulus. Therefore, the RV and RF are calculated as follows:

$$RV \text{ (ml)} = \text{Total stroke volume}$$
$$- \text{ systemic stroke volume}$$

$$RV \text{ (\%)} = (RV/\text{total stroke volume}) \times 100$$

Another approach to calculate RV and ERO is the proximal isovelocity surface area (PISA) method, which is based on the law of the conservation of mass (Fig. 2). The flow proximal to the regurgitant orifice is equal to the flow passing through the regurgitant orifice. Because the flow approaches the regurgitant orifice in hemispheres, the flow rate of these hemispheres is the product of the area of the hemisphere and the corresponding blood velocity. The blood velocity is the velocity at which aliasing occurs (Va) with color Doppler echocardiography. The area of the hemisphere is equal to $2pr^2$, where r is the radius of the hemisphere. Because the regurgitant flow is the same proximal to and through the regurgitant orifice, flow can be

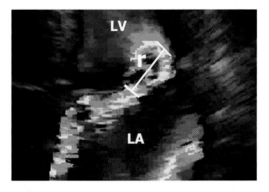

Fig. 2. Color flow recording of a MR jet—a zoomed view in the apical view. Color Doppler demonstrating severe mitral insufficiency caused by posterior leaflet prolapse. The severity of insufficiency is directly related to the radius (r) of the proximal flow convergence region. LA, left atrium; LV, left ventricle. (*From* Vannan MA, Liu Z, Rakowski H, et al, editors. Atlas of heart diseases: echocardiography. Philadelphia: Current Medicine LLC; 2005. © 2005, Current Medicine LLC; used with permission.)

calculated, and ERO and regurgitant volume can be derived as follows [18,21]:

$$ERO = (6.28 \times r^2 \times Va)/V\mathrm{max}$$

$$RV = ERO \times TVI$$

The PISA method performs comparably to other established invasive and noninvasive methods in the calculation of ERO and RV [19]. However, this method may lead to overestimation of ERO and RV in eccentric jets when the flow convergence is constrained. In patients who have mitral valve prolapse, phasic changes of MR occur. The effective orifice increases significantly from early to late systole, and regurgitant volume increases from early to mid-/late systole but decreases in late systole. In such cases, if the largest PISA value obtained is used indiscriminately, overestimation of the severity of the patient's MR ensues. No overestimation is observed, however, when the ERO that is calculated at the same time as the maximum regurgitant velocity is used [22]. Therefore, properly timed measurements, calculated by the PISA method, allow an accurate estimation of the overall ERO, even in this setting. A simplified measurement of proximal convergence has also been developed and is useful in most instances [23].

In one study, the authors prospectively evaluated 456 patients who had chronic MR using

quantitative MR techniques [24]. The investigators reported a mortality rate of 22% at 5 years. A major independent determinant of survival was the quantitative severity of the MR assessed by ERO. They found that patients who had a regurgitant orifice area ≥ 0.4 cm^2 had a 5-year survival rate of 58%, which was inferior to that of a matched control population (78%). Based on this data, the authors recommend that patients who have degenerative regurgitation and an ERO area of more than 40 mm^2 be considered promptly for surgery, regardless of the level of their symptoms or ventricular function [24]. Although the predictive value of the ERO appears to be high, caution is needed for several reasons as the authors generalize this approach. First, most previously established data apply to patients who have isolated primary MR. Therefore, patients who have mixed valve lesions, secondary MR, or left ventricular (LV) dysfunction are more complex. Second, quantitative evaluation of the severity of MR is time-consuming and technically demanding; accurate results depend on a meticulous approach by an experienced laboratory. Small errors in data-recording or measurement lead to large calculation errors in the ERO. Finally, echocardiogrphic evaluation of the severity of regurgitation should integrate several anatomical and Doppler variables; reliance on a single measure for clinical variables should be reassessed at more than one time to ensure accurate data [25].

Assessment of the consequences of mitral regurgitation

Left ventricular function

LV function is a powerful predictor of the postoperative outcomes of patients who have chronic MR. Patient survival after surgical correction of MR is dependent on the patient's preoperative LVEF [26]. In a study of 10-year survival after surgical correction of MR in patients at the Mayo Clinic, the survival rate with a preoperative LVEF of $\geq 60\%$ was similar to that expected for a population within the same age range (72% $\pm$ 4%). In contrast, the 10-year survival rate was poor for patients with LVEF $<50\%$ (32% $\pm$ 12%) [26]. Even a borderline LVEF (50%–60%) is associated with excess late mortality [41]. Increased LV size and decreased LVEF are markers of overt LV dysfunction. Unexpected postoperative LV dysfunction can occur, however, despite successful surgery. Therefore, LVEF and LV size are not precise indicators of LV dysfunction and fail to detect early LV contractile dysfunction. Variables that are noted to be more sensitive than LVEF in detecting early myocardial dysfunction in patients who have chronic MR include end-systolic volume indexed for body surface area and end-systolic dimensions measured by M-mode from the parasternal long axis window. The cutoff value for end-systolic dimension is 4.5 cm [27]. Diameter that is guided by M-mode is used for the assessment of LV size [26] and is very useful for diagnosing LV dilation, but it is less accurate for assessing LV size in the setting of LV dilation [28].

Stress echocardiography is a useful adjunct to clinical and Doppler echocardiographic testing when following up patients who have MR, especially in those patients in whom there is a concern that symptoms may be occurring or when the left ventricular size or function is approaching the end points at which surgery is recommended [29]. The addition of the stress component allows evaluation of other parameters of interest, such as pulmonary artery systolic pressure at peak exercise, functional capacity, and the response of the left ventricle to exercise (ie, the "contractile reserve"). A reduction in end-systolic volume at peak exercise (versus volume at rest), and an improvement in ejection fraction at peak were better predictors of LV function postoperatively than the preoperative resting ejection fraction. A recent study indicated that when contractile reserve is absent in patients who have chronic MR (ie, when there is a failure of LV function to improve with exercise or LV end-systolic volume to decrease), the patients tend to demonstrate progressive LV dysfunction when treated medically, which persists after corrective surgery in 20% of patients [30].

Left atrial size

In patients who have chronic MR, the left atrium (LA) dilates to accommodate the regurgitant volume without increasing atrial or pulmonary pressure. Whether LA size is a preoperative predictor of postoperative mortality is the source of some controversy. Although one study suggested that the LA size index was an independent predictor of death, this was only the case in patients with LVEF >75% (such patients have an excellent outlook anyway). Furthermore, other studies have failed to reproduce this finding. Some recent data have been produced which demonstrate that

preoperative LA size may be a preoperative predictor of postoperative morbidity [31,32].

Current guidelines for surgical interventions in mitral regurgitation and unresolved issues

Current guidelines (originally published in 1998) suggest surgical intervention in patients who have severe MR if there are significant symptoms, or at the onset of signs of LV dysfunction that have previously been shown to adversely affect outcome, such as an ejection fraction of <60% or significant LV dilatation with an end-systolic dimension of ≥45 mm². The guidelines stress the importance of using mitral valve repair for the correction of MR when feasible, and, in general, they suggest a lower threshold to intervene surgically when mitral valve repair appears both feasible and likely. The guidelines also suggest that surgery may be indicated even in the absence of symptoms or signs of LV dysfunction when atrial fibrillation ensues, or when pulmonary pressures are elevated to >50 mm Hg at rest or >60 mm Hg on exercise. The guidelines suggest that surgery is not generally indicated in asymptomatic patients with preserved LV function, even if mitral valve repair is feasible [27,33].

Early intervention in chronic MR is an ongoing debate, but echocardiography may help to resolve some of the questions. First, the clinician needs to be sure that earlier intervention results in better long-term outcomes than watchful waiting with prompt intervention based on conventional indications for surgery. A key factor in this decision is the likelihood that the valve can be repaired rather than replaced, a judgment that can be made by experienced echocardiographers [34,35]. In a patient with a valve that can be repaired and a low expected perioperative risk of complications or death, earlier intervention might be reasonable. However, if valve replacement is likely to be needed or if the surgical risk is higher, the balance shifts toward watchful waiting. The ideal next step should be a prospective, randomized clinical study of early surgery that is compared with surgery for conventional indications in patients who have severe asymptomatic MR, which is defined on the basis of the ERO area.

The decision to recommend surgery for an asymptomatic patient is always difficult; current guidelines are based on incomplete natural history data and on the consensus of experts, rather than on prospective randomized trials. The timing of mitral surgery often translates into a categorical answer when the patient is seen (ie, should the patient be advised to have mitral surgery promptly, or should the clinician advise follow-up with conservative management?). This process can be stratified according to the cause and severity of MR. Patients who have severe MR with overt severe consequences should be offered surgery, even in relatively high-risk patients and regardless of the repairability of the mitral valve. Although surgery performed with this type of presentation results in symptomatic improvement, it is associated with notable excess postoperative risk [26,36], but the postoperative outcome is far better than the outcome under medical treatment [37]. Some events that occur just prior to the visit are a strong incentive to propose surgery in a patient who has severe MR but neither overt symptoms nor LV dysfunction irrespective of repairability; these events are artial fibrillation; even paroxysmal; ventricular tachycardia at rest

or during exercise; or the observation of pulmonary hypertension by echocardiography [33]. With low probability of repair, patients are usually not referred to surgery if there are no clinical risk factors. With high probability of valve repair, the current guidelines [33] have become much more aggressive toward surgery—even if there are no symptoms or signs of LV dysfunction—if the operative risk is low. This aggressive approach will require a randomized clinical trial in the future to define the magnitude of its benefit. For regurgitant volumes measuring 45–60 mL/beat, there is usually no need for immediate surgery, but in certain rare circumstances, mitral surgery may be indicated. These circumstances involve valves that are repairable and patients who need a cardiac operation for a Maze procedure, bypass surgery, or another valve operation. In some patients with mitral valve prolapse and ventricular tachycardia at rest or with exertion, the authors

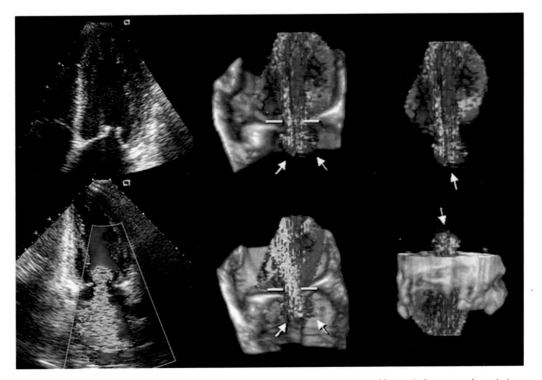

Fig. 3. Three-dimensional echocardiography images of MR. The left panels (*top and bottom*) show transthoracic imaging of thickened, restricted mitral valve with severe regurgitation. The middle panels (*top and bottom*) show three-dimensional regurgitant jet and spatial location and extent in two different orientations. Also observe that the proximal isovelocity surface area (PISA) (*arrows*) and vena contracta (*lines*) are of different dimensions in these two orientations. The right panels (*top and bottom*) show the shape of PISA: a three-dimensional color Doppler only in the upper figure and PISA seen from the left ventricle in the bottom (*arrows*). This case exemplifies the classic hemispheric geometry of PISA. (*From* Vannan MA, Liu Z, Rakowski H, et al, editors. Atlas of heart diseases: echocardiography. Philadelphia: Current Medicine LLC; 2005. © 2005, Current Medicine LLC; used with permission.)

have advised a mitral valve repair to suppress the volume overload. The comparison of a surgical approach to medical treatment and even the determination of the benefit of medical treatment under those circumstances remains to be defined [33]. Certainly, patients with an ERO of 40 mm^2 or more should be monitored more closely. In addition, the clinician may wish to offer selected patients earlier intervention after discussing the expected clinical outcomes, considering the effects of coexisting conditions, and weighing the patients' preferences [25]. Assessment of ERO or RV by quantitative echocardiography is technically demanding and requires considerable skill and practice if meaningful and reproducible results are to be obtained [17]. It is imperative that the accuracy and reproducibility of the quantitative parameters are established in each laboratory if echocardiography is to play a role in decision-making of asymptomatic chronic severe MR [38].

Future direction

Early detection of LV dysfunction and quantification of the exact amount of MR are crucial to managing chronic, severe MR. Therefore, more accurate information about mitral valve geometry, pathology and severity, and LV function is needed. Recent advances in echocardiography, such as Doppler tissue imaging and three-dimensional (3D) echocardiography, allow early detection of impaired LV function and provide more precise information about the severity of MR and mitral valve geometry.

Strain rate (SR) imaging is a relatively new technique that estimates spatial gradients in myocardial velocities and allows accurate quantification of regional myocardial function [39]. The translation or pathologic tethering to adjacent myocardial segments, which influence myocardial velocity measurements, does not influence SR imaging. Lee and colleagues demonstrate that the evaluation of global long-axis function by SR imaging is a feasible method for detecting subclinical LV dysfunction and can accurately predict contractile reserve in asymptomatic patients who have severe MR [40].

The assessment of the morphology, function, and pathology of the heart, and especially the mitral valve apparatus, by 3D echocardiography is more accurate in comparison to two-dimensional (2D) echocardiography. 3D echocardiography offers advantages for the morphologic and quantitative assessment of MR. It appears that 3D echocardiography has the potential for planning operations and assessing interventional or surgical results. Furthermore, 3D echocardiography may provide new quantitative indices that are unobtainable by conventional 2D imaging (Fig. 3). Both technical improvement and larger studies will enhance the clinical applicability of Doppler tissue imaging and 3D echocardiography in the near future [41].

Summary

Assessment and management of mitral valve regurgitation is a challenging clinical problem. Echocardiography is exceptionally sensitive for the detection of MR. Moreover, quantitation of the severity of the disease and the hemodynamic state are determined accurately by echocardiography. Information obtained by echocardiography is crucial to planning mitral replacement or repair. The development of newer technologies offers further refinement of echocardiographic assessment of patients who have MR.

References

[1] Otto CM. Timing of surgery in mitral regurgitation. Heart 2003;89(1):100–5.

[2] Thomson HL, Enriquez-Sarano M, Tajik AJ. Timing of surgery in patients with chronic, severe mitral regurgitation. Cardiol Rev 2001;9(3):137–43.

[3] Enriquez-Sarano M. Timing of mitral valve surgery. Heart 2002;87(1):79–85.

[4] Thomson HL, Enriquez-Sarano M. Echocardiographic assessment of mitral regurgitation. Cardiol Rev 2001;9(4):210–6.

[5] Sarano M, Schaff H, Tajik A, et al. Chronic mitral regurgitation. Philadelphia: Lippincott Williams & Wilkins; 2000.

[6] Freeman WK, Schaff HV, Khandheria BK, et al. Intraoperative evaluation of mitral valve regurgitation and repair by transesophageal echocardiography: incidence and significance of systolic anterior motion. J Am Coll Cardiol 1992;20:599–609.

[7] Hall SA, Brickner ME, Willett DL, et al. Assessment of mitral regurgitation severity by Doppler color flow mapping of the vena contracta. Circulation 1997;95:636–42.

[8] Mele D, Vandervoort P, Palacios I, et al. Proximal jet size by Doppler color flow mapping predicts severity of mitral regurgitation: clinical studies. Circulation 1995;91:746–54.

[9] Baumgartner H, Schima H, Kuhn P. Value and limitations of proximal jet dimensions for the quantitation of valvular regurgitation: an in vitro study using Doppler flow imaging. J Am Soc Echocardiogr 1991; 4:57–66.

[10] Klein AL, Obarski TP, Stewart WJ, et al. Transesophageal Doppler echocardiography of pulmonary venous flow: a new marker of mitral regurgitation severity. J Am Coll Cardiol 1991;18:518–26.

[11] Nagueh SF. Assessment of valvular regurgitation with Doppler echocardiography. Cardiol Clin 1998; 16:405–19.

[12] Griffin BP. Timing of surgical intervention in chronic mitral regurgitation: is vigilance enough? Circulation 2006;113(18):2169–72.

[13] Spain MG, Smith MD, Grayburn PA, et al. Quantitative assessment of mitral regurgitation by Doppler color flow imaging: angiographic and hemodynamic correlations. J Am Coll Cardiol 1989; 13:585–90.

[14] Sahn DJ. Instrumentation and physical factors related to visualization of stenotic and regurgitant jets by Doppler color flow mapping. J Am Coll Cardiol 1988;12:1354–65.

[15] Enriquez-Sarano M, Dujardin KS, Tribouilloy CM, et al. Determinants of pulmonary venous flow reversal in mitral regurgitation and its usefulness in determining the severity of regurgitation. Am J Cardiol 1999;83:535–41.

[16] Enriquez-Sarano M, Bailey KR, Seward JB, et al. Quantitative Doppler assessment of valvular regurgitation. Circulation 1993;87:841–8.

[17] Zoghbi WA, Enriquez-Sarano M, Foster B, et al. Recommendations for evaluation of the severity of native valvular regurgitation with two dimensional and Doppler echocardiography. J Am Soc Echocardiogr 2003;16:777–802.

[18] Enriquez-Sarano M, Seward JB, Bailey KR, et al. Effective regurgitant orifice area: a noninvasive Doppler development of an old hemodynamic concept. J Am Coll Cardiol 1994;23:443–51.

[19] Enriquez-Sarano M, Miller FA, Hayes SN, et al. Effective mitral regurgitant orifice area: clinical use and pitfalls of the proximal isovelocity surface area method. J Am Coll Cardiol 1995;25:703–9.

[20] Dujardin KS, Enriquez-Sarano M, Bailey KR, et al. Grading of mitral regurgitation by quantitative Doppler echocardiography: calibration by left ventricular angiography in routine clinical practice. Circulation 1997;96:3409–15.

[21] Vandervoort PM, Rivera JM, Mele D, et al. Application of color Doppler flow mapping to calculate effective regurgitant orifice area. An in vitro study and initial clinical observations. Circulation 1993; 88:1150–6.

[22] Enriquez-Sarano M, Sinak LJ, Tajik AJ, et al. Changes in effective regurgitant orifice throughout systole in patients with mitral valve prolapse. A clinical study using the proximal isovelocity surface area method. Circulation 1995;92:2951–8.

[23] Rossi A, Dujardin KS, Bailey KR, et al. Rapid estimation of regurgitant volume by the proximal isovelocity surface area method in mitral regurgitation: can continuous-wave Doppler

echocardiography be omitted? J Am Soc Echocardiogr 1998;11:138–48.

[24] Enriquez-Sarano M, Avierinos JF, Messika-Zeitoun D, et al. Quantitative determinants of the outcome of asymptomatic mitral regurgitation. N Engl J Med 2005;352:875–83.

[25] Otto CM. Evaluation and management of chronic mitral regurgitation. N Engl J Med 2001;345:740–6.

[26] Enriquez-Sarano M, Tajik AJ, Schaff HV, et al. Echocardiographic prediction of survival after surgical correction of organic mitral regurgitation. Circulation 1994;90:830–7.

[27] Bonow R, Carabello B, DeLeon A, et al. ACC/AHA guidelines for the management of patients with valvular heart disease. Circulation 1998;98: 1949–84.

[28] Dujardin KS, Enriquez-Sarano M, Rossi A, et al. Echocardiographic assessment of left ventricular remodeling: are left ventricular diameters suitable tools? J Am Coll Cardiol 1997;30:1534–41.

[29] Leung D, Griffin BP, Stewart W, et al. Left ventricular function after valve repair for chronic mitral regurgitation: predictive value of preoperative assessment of contractile reserve by exercise echocardiography. J Am Coll Cardiol 1996;28: 1198–205.

[30] Lee R, Haluska B, Leung DY, et al. Functional and prognostic implications of left ventricular contractile reserve in patients with asymptomatic severe mitral regurgitation. Heart 2005;91:1407–12.

[31] Chua YL, Schaff HV, Orszulak TA, et al. Outcome of mitral valve repair in patients with preoperative atrial fibrillation. Should the maze procedure be combined with mitral valvuloplasty? J Thorac Cardiovasc Surg 1994;107:408–15.

[32] Avierinos J, Sarano M. Long-term outcome of mitral valve prolapse in the population: is mitral valve prolapse uniformly benign? [abstract]. J Am Soc Echocardiogr 2000;13:504.

[33] Bonow RO, Carabello BA, Kanu C, et al. ACC/AHA 2006 guidelines for the management of patients with valvular heart disease: a report of the American College of Cardiology/American Heart Association Task Force on Practice Guidelines (writing committee to revise the 1998 guidelines for the management of patients with valvular heart disease): developed in collaboration with the Society of Cardiovascular Anesthesiologists: endorsed by the Society for Cardiovascular Angiography and Interventions and the Society of Thoracic Surgeons. Circulation 2006;114(5):e84–231.

[34] Ling LH, Enriquez-Sarano M, Seward JB, et al. Early surgery in patients with mitral regurgitation due to flail leaflets: a long-term outcome study. Circulation 1997;96:1819–25.

[35] Rosenhek R, Rader F, Klaar U, Gabriel H, et al. Outcome of watchful waiting in asymptomatic severe mitral regurgitation. Circulation 2006;113(18): 2238–44.

[36] Tribouilloy C, Enriquez-Sarano M, Schaff H, et al. Impact of preoperative symptoms on survival after surgical correction of organic mitral regurgitation: rationale for optimizing surgical indications. Circulation 1999;99:400–5.

[37] Ling H, Enriquez-Sarano M, Seward J, et al. Clinical outcome of mitral regurgitation due to flail leaflets. N Engl J Med 1996;335:1417–23.

[38] Bridgewater B, Hooper T, Munsch C, et al. Mitral repair best practice: proposed standards. Heart 2006; 92(7):939–44.

[39] Heimdal A, Stoylen A, Torp H, et al. Real-time strain rate imaging of the left ventricle by ultrasound. J Am Soc Echocardiogr 1998;11:1013–9.

[40] Lee R, Hanekom L, Marwick TH, et al. Prediction of subclinical left ventricular dysfunction with strain rate imaging in patients with asymptomatic severe mitral regurgitation. Am J Cardiol 2004;94(10): 1333–7.

[41] Valocik G, Kamp O, Visser CA. Three-dimensional echocardiography in mitral valve disease. Eur J Echocardiogr 2005;6(6):443–54.

Heart Failure Clin 2 (2006) 435–442

Aortic Stenosis: From Pressure Overload to Heart Failure

Blase A. Carabello, MD[a,b,*]

[a]*Baylor College of Medicine, Houston, TX, USA*
[b]*Veterans Affairs Medical Center, Houston, TX, USA*

In 1973, Grossman and colleagues [1] postulated that pressure overload increased systolic wall stress, which became the putative signal to start the cascade of events leading to concentric left ventricular hypertrophy (LVH) (Fig. 1). Stress (σ) is defined by the Laplace equation, where $\sigma = P \times R/2h$, and P = left ventricular (LV) pressure, R = LV radius, and h = LV thickness. Thus, in this schema, as the pressure term increases in the numerator, it can be offset by concomitant increases in the thickness term in the denominator. Because stress is a good approximation of afterload, and because afterload is a key determinant of ejection performance, normalization of afterload is believed to be a compensatory mechanism that helps to maintain cardiac output in the face of hemodynamic overload. Unfortunately, the compensatory nature of hypertrophy is not so clear-cut. In many cases, hypertrophy is associated with pathologic consequences; in others, the hypertrophy is not adequate to normalize wall stress or is so abundant as to "overcompensate" for the overload [2–5]. This article discusses the regulation of cardiac growth in response to an overload, the mechanisms by which LVH becomes pathologic, the transition to heart failure, and current management options.

Myocardial growth regulation

Although recent evidence demonstrates that myocyte replication can occur at a low rate in adults [6], it is generally held that most myocytes are terminally differentiated, so that cardiac growth occurs primarily from hypertrophy of existing myocytes, rather than by hyperplasia. Thus, hypertrophy is a necessary mechanism for allowing the heart of an infant to grow 20-fold to meet the circulatory demands of the adult. Such hypertrophy obviously is physiologic. Additionally, athletes who are engaged in isometric and isotonic exercise develop extensive concentric and eccentric LVH, respectively. Studies of systolic and diastolic function in athletes almost universally demonstrate normal function [7–10]. In contrast, similar amounts of LVH arising from disease states, such as valvular heart disease or hypertension, usually are attended by systolic dysfunction, diastolic dysfunction, or both. Thus, differences between physiologic and pathologic hypertrophy must encompass more than just magnitude. Presumably, a key difference between the two conditions in some way reflects the intermittent overloads that are experienced by athletes who inevitably rest versus the pathologic overloads (eg, aortic stenosis [AS]), where the overload is constant and unremitting.

The paradigm presented in Fig. 1 suggests a feedback loop wherein stress induces hypertrophy; this, in turn, normalizes stress and turns the hypertrophic process off. In theory, just enough hypertrophy should develop to normalize stress. Indeed, this often is the case; however, there are many examples where inadequate hypertrophy develops, stress (afterload) is increased, and ejection performance is reduced [3,4,11]. In other cases, hypertrophy seems excessive, stress is subnormal, and ejection fraction is greater than normal. This seems especially true in children and elderly women who have AS [5,12]. The question arises

---

* Veterans Affairs Medical Center, 1 Baylor Plaza, Building 100, Room 4C211, Houston, TX 77030-4211.
E-mail address: blaseanthony.carabello@med.va.gov

1551-7136/06/$ - see front matter © 2007 Elsevier Inc. All rights reserved.
doi:10.1016/j.hfc.2006.11.001

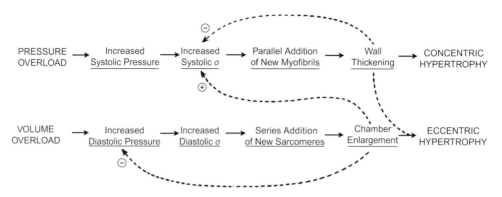

Fig. 1. A feedback loop is demonstrated where the increased systolic stress of pressure overload leads to sarcomere replication in parallel causing concentric LVH, whereas increased diastolic stress leads to parallel sarcomere replication and eccentric hypertrophy. (*Data from* Grossman W, Jones D, McLaurin LP. Wall stress and patterns of hypertrophy in the human left ventricle. J Clin Invest 1975;53:332–41.)

as to whether these varying degrees of hypertrophy occur from differences in the disease itself (ie, the severity of stenosis or the rapidity with which it develops), or whether the differences in hypertrophy represent differences in an individual's response to a similar overload. To address this issue, Koide and colleagues [2] created a model of gradually developing canine AS, in which an externally regulated band created a similar pressure load in the experimental subjects. As shown in Fig. 2, some dogs developed marked hypertrophy, whereas others developed much less hypertrophy in response to the same overload. As shown in Fig. 3, the dogs who had only modest hypertrophy had higher wall stress even before banding, and never developed enough hypertrophy to normalize stress. Thus, the two groups of dogs responded differently to the same stimulus to hypertrophy, suggesting downstream modulation of the mechanism by which the mechanical stimulus was transduced into a growth response. It is likely that this modulation revolves around differences in the multiple downstream signaling pathways that lead to hypertrophy. This response in dogs is similar to the variable response seen in man, in terms of the compensatory versus noncompensatory hypertrophy that develops in response to AS.

Hypertrophy and systolic dysfunction in aortic stenosis

Fig. 4 demonstrates the two basic mechanisms that are responsible for systolic failure in AS. In this group of 14 patients, all had reduced ejection fraction and clinical heart failure [11]. One group

had reduced ejection fraction that was due to afterload excess. In these patients, hypertrophy was inadequate to normalize wall stress, so increased stress caused reduced ejection fraction. This group had dramatic clinical improvement following aortic valve replacement wherein

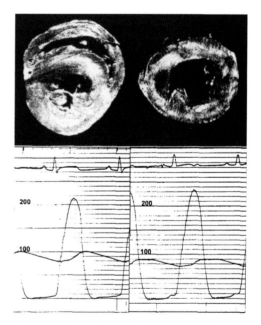

Fig. 2. In this experimental model of AS, similar pressure overload resulted in severe LVH (*left panel*) in some dogs, but only modest LVH (*right panel*) in others. (*From* Koide M, Nagatsu M, Zile MR, et al. Premorbid determinants of left ventricular dysfunction in a novel mode of gradually induced pressure overload in the adult canine. Circulation 1997;95(6):1349–51; with permission.)

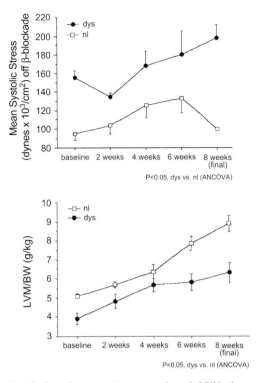

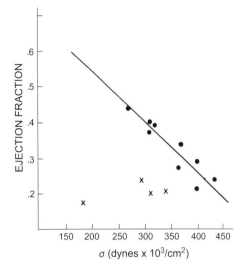

Fig. 4. The wall stress–ejection fraction relationship for two groups of patients who had AS who had heart failure and systolic dysfunction. Patients with a good outcome following surgery (*filled circles*) had reduced ejection fraction because of afterload mismatch, whereas patients with a poor outcome (*Xs*) had ejection fraction reduction that was not caused by afterload mismatch alone, indicating myocardial dysfunction. (*From* Carabello BA, Green LH, Grossman W, et al. Hemodynamic determinants of prognosis of aortic valve replacement in critical aortic stenosis and advanced congestive heart failure. Circulation 1980;62:46; with permission.)

Fig. 3. Systolic stress (*upper panel*) and LVH (*lower panel*) for dogs who had AS that developed only modest LVH and LV dysfunction (*filled circles*) versus dogs that developed severe LVH but had normal systolic function (*open circles*). Throughout and even before banding, the group with modest LVH always had higher stress, yet less hypertrophy; this suggested a different transduction of the putative signal for LVH (stress) into myocardial growth between the two groups of dogs. BW, body weight; dys, dysfunction; LVM, LV mass; nl, normal. (*From* Koide M, Nagatsu M, Zile MR, et al. Premorbid determinants of left ventricular dysfunction in a novel mode of gradually induced pressure overload in the adult canine. Circulation 1997;95(6):1349–51; with permission.)

afterload was reduced, ejection fraction improved, and heart failure abated. In the second group, ejection fraction was reduced out of proportion to the afterload excess, indicating a contractile deficit. This group failed to respond to aortic valve replacement. Obviously, this raises the question of what causes contractile dysfunction in AS. Indeed, the mechanisms that produce the transition from hypertrophy to failure have long been sought, and no unified hypothesis is accepted widely. It is probable that multiple mechanisms are responsible for the contractile deficit in some patients who have AS.

Ischemia

In normal subjects, increased myocardial oxygen demand is met by increased coronary blood flow that can increase by up to eight-fold [13]; however, in subjects who have concentric LHV, flow reserve is diminished to twofold to threefold. Further, in normal subjects, endocardial flow exceeds epicardial flow by about 20%, which accommodates the increased endocardial oxygen demand [14,15]; however, in concentric LVH, this preferential flow to the endocardium is reversed, which may lead to subendocardial ischemia. Indeed, increased demand caused by atrial pacing does cause endocardial dysfunction [16]. Thus, the contractile dysfunction that is seen in patients who have AS during exercise probably is explained, in part, by evoked subendocardial ischemia. Further, although not proven, it is conceivable that repeated episodes of ischemia lead to myocardial stunning and more persistent dysfunction, even at rest.

Calcium handling

Calcium is the prime regulator of contractility in all mammalian hearts. Thus, it is reasonable to expect that abnormalities in calcium handling might be responsible for contractile abnormalities in AS. In almost all types of hypertrophy [17], there is down-regulation in SERCA 2, the system that returns calcium back to the sarcoplasmic reticulum following contraction. A deficit in calcium return means that less calcium is available for release during the next contraction, which reduces contractility. SERCA 2 is depressed even before contractility is reduced, however, which makes it more difficult to prove that SERCA 2 depression is responsible for the transition from LVH to LVH with failure.

Fibrosis

As hypertrophy progresses, the percentage of the myocardium that is made up of noncontractile elements, such as collagen, increases. Increased collagen is associated with contractile element loss; therefore, fibrosis also contributes to the contractile deficit that is seen in some patients who have AS.

Cytoskeletal abnormalities

Tsutsui and colleagues [18] noted that in AS with high wall stress and inadequate hypertrophy, tubulin—which forms the microtubular components of the cytoskeleton—is increased greatly, as are the microtubules themselves. Increased density of the cytoskeleton acts as an internal stent that prevents the contractile elements from shortening, which, in turn, impairs contraction.

Hypertrophy and diastolic dysfunction in aortic stenosis

Diastolic function is clearly abnormal in many patients who have AS, and it contributes to the overall picture of heart failure [19]. Usually, diastole is divided into active relaxation and passive filling; both elements can be abnormal in patients who have AS [20]. Active relaxation is defined as the period when calcium is pumped back into the sarcoplasmic reticulum, and which causes the interaction between the contractile proteins to diminish greatly. In the cardiac cycle, it takes place between aortic valve closure and mitral valve opening. As shown in Fig. 5, the pressure decay following aortic valve closure in patients who have AS is slowed; this indicates impairment of

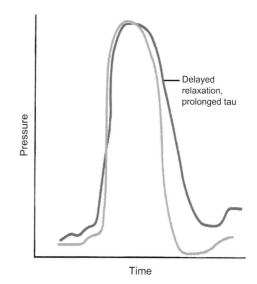

Fig. 5. Delayed relaxation is inferred from the slowing of the fall in ventricular pressure during isovolumic diastole. (*From* Carroll JD, Hess OM. Assessment of normal and abnormal cardiac function. In: Zipes D, Libby P, Bonow R, et al, editors. Braunwald's heart disease: a textbook of cardiovascular medicine. Philadelphia: Saunders; 2005. p. 498; with permission.)

active relaxation because of persistent contractile protein interaction [21]. In turn, slowed active relaxation delays opening of the mitral valve and reduces diastolic filling time.

Following mitral valve opening, the pressure–volume relationship of the left ventricle in AS is shifted upward and to the left, which indicates increased ventricular stiffness. As such, a greater filling pressure is required to achieve any filling volume. Higher filling pressure, in turn, leads to pulmonary congestion and the signs and symptoms of heart failure. Increased ventricular stiffness stems from increased wall thickness. It is harder to fill a thick-walled structure than a thin-walled one. In addition, increased collagen elements that develop in advanced disease make the myocardium itself stiffer, which impairs LV filling further.

Clinical consequences of hypertrophy and failure

Fig. 6 demonstrates the natural history of AS according to symptom status. Once angina has developed, the average survival time without aortic valve replacement (AVR) is about 5 years [22]. Survival averages 3 years after the onset of syncope, whereas the onset of heart failure presages the worst prognosis, with an average survival

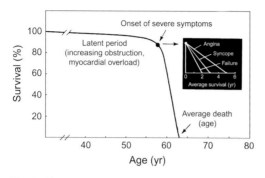

Fig. 6. The natural history of AS. There is a long latent period where survival is nearly normal; however, once the symptoms of angina, syncope, and heart failure develop, survival plummets, with the symptoms of heart failure presaging the worst prognosis. (*From* Ross J Jr, Braunwald E. Aortic stenosis. Circulation 1968;38:62; with permission.)

of only 2 years after symptom onset. Patients with depressed ejection fraction have a dramatic response to AVR if their depressed performance was predicated upon afterload excess and a large transvalvular gradient. In such cases, AVR immediately relieves obstruction to outflow, afterload decreases, and ejection fraction and cardiac output improve rapidly (Fig. 7) [23].

The opposite is true for patients with a low gradient and low ejection fraction where contractile dysfunction now plays a major role in the observed LV dysfunction. Contractile dysfunction may or may not improve following surgery and if it does improve, the process is gradual rather than immediate. For this reason, virtually every study of low ejection fraction low gradient AS patients has found increased operative mortality, less postoperative improvement in cardiac performance and a worse overall prognosis than other AS patients [11,24–26]. Yet, some such subjects do improve dramatically following AVR [23–25]. Thus, management of these patients is quite problematic and much work has been done in an attempt to better define which of these patients is likely to benefit from surgery versus those for which conservative management is more appropriate.

Separating true stenosis from pseudoaortic stenosis

It is generally held that if LV dysfunction has been caused by severe AS, relief of the obstruction should lead to hemodynamic improvement. Unfortunately, it may be difficult to discern when severe AS is present in the face of severe LV

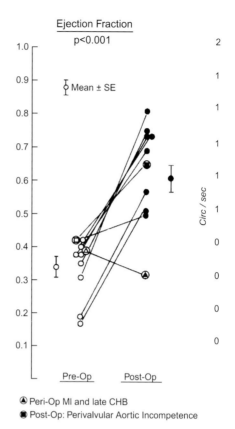

⊕ Peri-Op MI and late CHB
● Post-Op: Perivalvular Aortic Incompetence

Fig. 7. Reduced preoperative ejection fraction in patients who have AS improves dramatically following AVR when preoperative afterload is increased. CHB, complete heart block; Circ, circumferences; MI, myocardial infarction. (*From* Smith N, McAnulty JH, Rahimtoola SH. Severe aortic stenosis with impaired left ventricular function and clinical heart failure: results of valve replacement. Circulation 1978;58(2):261; with permission.)

dysfunction. A small calculated valve area can stem from two causes. First, severe AS may cause severely reduced cardiac output. Conversely, a ventricle damaged from coronary disease or a primary cardiomyopathy might be unable to open an only mildly or moderately diseased aortic valve (pseudo-AS). In both cases, the valve area is calculated to be small, at least at rest. One technique for distinguishing true AS from pseudo-AS is to increase the force of LV contraction and cardiac output with administration of an inotrope or a vasodilator [26,27]. Calculated valve area is flow dependent at low flows. In pseudo-AS, however, increasing flow causes a much greater increase in flow than gradient; this causes a large increase in aortic valve area (AVA) compared with true AS, where output and gradient increase in tandem. Examples are shown in Table 1. If output increases toward 5 L/min, but AVA increases less than 0.3 cm^2 and AVA is still less than 1.0 cm^2, it is probable that true AS is present; this premise is strengthened by finding heavy calcification of the aortic valve. It is presumed that correction of true AS should benefit the patient, whereas correction of pseudo-AS should not. Although logical, no studies have compared the effects of AVR in true AS versus pseudo-AS. It is conceivable that even relief of mild to moderate AS could benefit the severely myopathic LV.

Inotropic reserve

As shown in Fig. 8, patients with low gradient and low ejection fraction have a poor prognosis, with a roughly 25% operative mortality and only a 50% 4-year survival. Fig. 9 shows that following AVR, ejection fraction improves only modestly in this group of patients, with the notable exception that there is dramatic postoperative improvement in some patients [25]. Perhaps the best way to prognosticate outcome in this group of patients is to examine their response to inotropic infusion. Monin and colleagues [28] reported the surgical outcome of AS patients with low gradient and low ejection fraction, with respect to their response to dobutamine infusion (Fig. 10). Group I had at least a 20% increase in stroke volume with dobutamine infusion. Group II failed to have inotropic reserve. Operative mortality was about 10% in group I, and triple that (~30%) in group II. Group I also had better long-term survival. Still challenging is the fact that despite a high operative risk, group II faired better with AVR than with medical therapy. Indeed, the same investigators reported that many patients in group II who survived surgery had significant improvement following AVR [29].

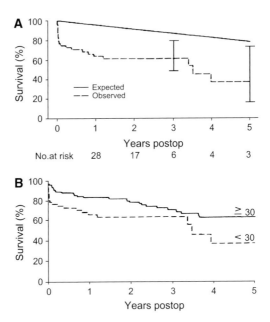

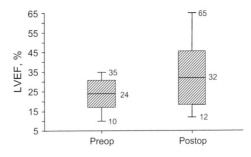

Fig. 8. Survival following AVR for patients with low ejection fraction and low gradient. High operative risk and poor overall survival is demonstrated. (*From* Connolly HM, Oh JK, Schaff HV, et al. Severe aortic stenosis with low transvalvular gradient and severe left ventricular dysfunction: result of aortic valve replacement in 52 patients. Circulation 2000;101:1943; with permission.)

One caveat is that in the patient who has AS and coronary disease, inotropic stimulation could induce ischemia, leading to the false conclusion that inotropic reserve was absent, when, in fact, induced ischemia prevented it from occurring.

Fig. 9. Preoperative and postoperative ejection fraction for the patients shown in Fig. 8. Ejection fraction improved only modestly compared with that seen in Fig. 6, although some patients had dramatic improvement. (*From* Connolly HM, Oh JK, Schaff HV, et al. Severe aortic stenosis with low transvalvular gradient and severe left ventricular dysfunction: result of aortic valve replacement in 52 patients. Circulation 2000;101:1943; with permission.)

Table 1
True versus pseudo-aortic stenosis

	True AS		Pseudo-AS	
	Rest	Dobutamine	Rest	Dobutamine
CO L/min	3.5	5.0	3.5	5.0
Gradient mm Hg	25	40	25	25
AVA cm^2	0.7	0.8	0.7	1.0

Abbreviation: CO, cardiac output.

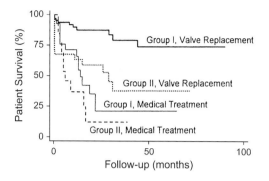

Fig. 10. Postoperative survival is shown for patients who have AS with low ejection fraction and low gradient who had increased stroke volume with dobutamine infusion (group I) versus those who failed to show inotropic reserve (group II). (*From* Monin JL, Quere JP, Monchi M, et al. Low-gradient aortic stenosis: operative risk stratification and predictors for long-term outcome: a multicenter study using dobutamine stress hemodynamics. Circulation 2003;108:322.)

Severe heart failure and nitroprusside

Conventional wisdom is that vasodilators should be avoided in severe AS, because the decrease in peripheral resistance that they cause cannot be met by an increase in cardiac output that is restricted by obstruction to outflow. Thus, resistance decreases and output remains the same, so that vasodilators are likely to cause hypotension and even syncope. Therefore, it is of extreme interest that in a recent report of carefully monitored nitroprusside infusion in AS patients who had pulmonary edema, substantial clinical improvement was noted [30]. Analysis of the mechanism of benefit showed that nitroprusside's salutary effects were not due to its reduction in peripheral resistance; rather, the drug acted to increase contractility [31]. Although unproven, it is likely that improvement following nitroprusside infusion reduced LV filling pressure. High filling pressure compresses the subendocardium, which reduces coronary blood flow to that layer of the heart, and, in turn, induces ischemic contractile dysfunction. By reducing filling pressure, it is likely that the drug improved subendocardial ischemia, and, thus, improved contractility.

Summary

The pressure overload that is caused by AS is compensated by LVH, a double-edged sword. Although LVH helps to maintain normal afterload on the left ventricle, properties of the concentrically hypertrophied LV are pathologic. These pathologic properties lead to systolic and diastolic LV dysfunction. When systolic dysfunction is due to afterload excess, improvement following AVR is dramatic and prognosis is good. When systolic dysfunction is mediated primarily by a contractile deficit, prognosis is considerably worse. Patients in this category who demonstrate inotropic reserve still have a mostly good outcome following surgery. Those without inotropic reserve have a much worse prognosis, although even some of these patients benefit from AVR. A remaining challenge is to detect, preoperatively, who in this last group of patients will benefit from AVR, even in the absence of inotropic reserve.

References

[1] Grossman W, Jones D, McLaurin LP. Wall stress and patterns of hypertrophy in the human left ventricle. J Clin Invest 1975;53:332–41.

[2] Koide M, Nagatsu M, Zile MR, et al. Premorbid determinants of left ventricular dysfunction in a novel mode of gradually induced pressure overload in the adult canine. Circulation 1997;95(6):1349–51.

[3] Gunther S, Grossman W. Determinants of ventricular function in pressure-overload hypertrophy in man. Circulation 1979;59:679–88.

[4] Huber D, Grimm J, Koch R, et al. Determinants of ejection performance in aortic stenosis. Circulation 1981;64:126–34.

[5] Donner R, Carabello BA, Black I, et al. Left ventricular wall stress in compensated aortic stenosis in children. Am J Cardiol 1983;51(6):946–51.

[6] Beltrami CA, Di Loreto C, Finato N, et al. Proliferating cell nuclear antigen (PCNA), DNA synthesis and mitosis in myocytes following cardiac transplantation in man. J Mol Cell Cardiol 1997;29:2789–802.

[7] Zoncu S, Pelliccia A, Mercuro G. Assessment of regional systolic and diastolic wall motion velocities in highly trained athletes by pulsed wave Doppler tissue imaging. J Am Soc Echocardiogr 2002;15(9):900–5.

[8] Schannwell CM, Schneppenheim M, Plehn G, et al. Left ventricular diastolic function in physiologic and pathologic hypertrophy. Am J Hypertens 2002;15(6):513–7.

[9] Vinereanu D, Florescu N, Sculthorpe N, et al. Differentiation between pathologic and physiologic left ventricular hypertrophy by tissue Doppler assessment of long-axis function in patients with hypertrophic cardiomyopathy or systemic hypertension and in athletes. Am J Cardiol 2001;88(1):53–8.

[10] Colan SD. Mechanics of left ventricular systolic and diastolic function in physiologic hypertrophy of the athlete's heart. Cardiol Clin 1997;15(3):355–72.

[11] Carabello BA, Green LH, Grossman W, et al. Hemodynamic determinants of prognosis of aortic valve replacement in critical aortic stenosis and advanced congestive heart failure. Circulation 1980; 62:42–8.

[12] Carroll JD, Carroll EP, Feldman T, et al. Sex-associated differences in left ventricular function in aortic stenosis of the elderly. Circulation 1992;86(4): 1099–107.

[13] Marcus ML, Doty DB, Hiratzka LF, et al. Decreased coronary reserve: a mechanism for angina pectoris in patients with aortic stenosis and normal coronary arteries. N Engl J Med 1982;307:1362–6.

[14] Rembert JC, Kleinman LH, Fedor JM, et al. Myocardial blood flow distribution in concentric left ventricular hypertrophy. J Clin Invest 1978;62:379.

[15] Bach RJ, Vrobel TR. Effects of exercise on blood flow in the hypertrophied heart. Am J Cardiol 1979; 44:1029.

[16] Nakano K, Corin WJ, Spann JF Jr, et al. Abnormal subendocardial blood flow in pressure overload hypertrophy is associated with pacing-induced subendocardial dysfunction. Circ Res 1989;65(6):1555–64.

[17] Ito K, Yan X, Feng X, et al. Transgenic expression of sarcoplasmic reticulum Ca(2 +) atpase modifies the transition from hypertrophy to early heart failure. Circ Res 2001;89:422–9.

[18] Tsutsui H, Oshihara K, Cooper GT. Cytoskeletal role in the contractile dysfunction of hypertrophied myocardium. Science 1993;260(5108):682–7.

[19] Hess OM, Ritter M, Schneider J, et al. Diastolic stiffness and myocardial structure in aortic valve disease before and after valve replacement. Circulation 1984; 69:855–65.

[20] Zile M, Brutsaert D. New concepts in diastolic dysfunction and diastolic heart failure II. Causal mechanisms and treatment. Circulation 2002;105:1503.

[21] Carroll JD, Hess OM. Assessment of normal and abnormal cardiac function. In: Zipes D, Libby P, Bonow R, et al, editors. Braunwald's heart disease: a textbook of cardiovascular medicine. Philadelphia: Saunders; 2005. p. 491–507.

[22] Ross J Jr, Braunwald E. Aortic stenosis. Circulation 1968;38:61–7.

[23] Smith N, McAnulty JH, Rahimtoola SH. Severe aortic stenosis with impaired left ventricular function and clinical heart failure: results of valve replacement. Circulation 1978;58(2):255–64.

[24] Brogan WC III, Grayburn PA, Lange RA, et al. Prognosis after valve replacement in patients with severe aortic stenosis and a low transvalvular pressure gradient. J Am Coll Cardiol 1993;21: 1657–60.

[25] Connolly HM, Oh JK, Schaff HV, et al. Severe aortic stenosis with low transvalvular gradient and severe left ventricular dysfunction: result of aortic valve replacement in 52 patients. Circulation 2000; 101:1940–6.

[26] Nishimura RA, Grantham JA, Connolly HM, et al. Low-output, low-gradient aortic stenosis in patients with depressed left ventricular systolic function: the clinical utility of the dobutamine challenge in the catheterization laboratory. Circulation 2002;106: 809–13.

[27] Cannon JD Jr, Zile MR, Crawford FA Jr, et al. Aortic valve resistance as an adjunct to the Gorlin formula in assessing the severity of aortic stenosis in symptomatic patients. J Am Coll Cardiol 1992; 20(7):1517–23.

[28] Monin JL, Quere JP, Monchi M, et al. Low-gradient aortic stenosis: operative risk stratification and predictors for long-term outcome: a multicenter study using dobutamine stress hemodynamics. Circulation 2003;108:319–24.

[29] Quere JP, Monin JL, Levy F, et al. Influence of preoperative left ventricular contractile reserve on postoperative ejection fraction in low-gradient aortic stenosis. Circulation 2006;113(14):1738–44.

[30] Khot UN, Novaro GM, Popovic ZB, et al. Nitroprusside in critically ill patients with left ventricular dysfunction and aortic stenosis. N Engl J Med 2005; 348(18):1756–63.

[31] Popovic ZB, Khot UN, Novaro GM, et al. Effects of sodium nitroprusside in aortic stenosis associated with severe heart failure: pressure-volume loop analysis using a numerical model. Am J Physiol Heart Circ Physiol 2005;288(1):H416–23.

**ELSEVIER
SAUNDERS**

Heart Failure Clin 2 (2006) 443–452

**HEART
FAILURE
CLINICS**

Left Ventricular Dysfunction and Mitral Stenosis

Andrew J.P. Klein, MD, John D. Carroll, MD*

University of Colorado Health Sciences, Denver, CO, USA

Rheumatic fever once dominated as the leading cause of valvular heart disease, and there has been a progressive decline in its prevalence over the last 50 years. Although any valves might be affected by rheumatic fever, the ones most often affected are the mitral and aortic valves. Mitral stenosis (MS) is the major valvular sequela of rheumatic fever observed in adults. Although there are numerous other causes of MS, including severe mitral annular calcification, carcinoid tumor, methylsergide therapy, Fabry's disease, Whipple's disease, systemic lupus erythematous, and mucopolysaccharidosis [1], more than 99% of MS is rheumatic in nature [2].

The prevalence of left ventricular (LV) dysfunction with MS is controversial. Much of the research performed on this topic is several decades old secondary to the declining prevalence of rheumatic heart disease. Although it is generally believed that LV contractility is normal in most cases of MS [3], some studies have suggested otherwise. Several studies have reported that the prevalence of a reduced LV ejection fraction in patients who have pure MS may be as high as 33% [4–7]. Most recently, Snyder and colleagues [8] reported an ejection fraction of 0.50 or less in 21 of 72 patients undergoing cardiac catheterization for MS. Choi and colleagues [9], using a radionucleotide technique, reported an ejection fraction of less than 0.45 in 18 of 36 patients who had MS.

Before the advent of surgical commisurotomy, the importance of determining the etiology of the

LV dysfunction was a moot point because there was no effective therapy for either problem. With the advent of surgical procedures and later endovascular therapies, it has become clinically relevant to assess the effect of valvular obstruction versus myocardial insufficiency in MS [10]. Studies by Harvey and colleagues [11] and Fleming and Wood [12] were the first of many that have sought to determine the cause and prevalence of LV dysfunction in MS. This article focuses on the leading mechanistic theories and proposed treatment modalities for patients who have LV dysfunction and MS.

To appreciate the attempts to explain how this valvular disorder might induce LV dysfunction, one must have an understanding of the pathophysiology of MS, which is extensively reviewed elsewhere in this issue. The essential mechanisms to be noted are the pancardiac inflammation that occurs during acute rheumatic fever and the effects of potential chronic inflammation on the myocardium. During the acute phase, all three layers of the heart are involved (endocardium, myocardium, and pericardium) [3]. Although the most common long-term effect of this acute inflammation is valvular scarring and stenosis, chronic inflammation and scarring of the endocardium may occur long after the initial acute attack. The continuum between acute and chronic inflammation is represented histologically by initial fibroid necrosis, which is followed by the appearance of histiocytes and giant cells in a granulomatous stage [13]. This chronic inflammation with resultant fibrosis may be one feature of the so-called "myocardial factor" noted by Fleming and Wood [12].

In addition to the primary myocardial effects of rheumatic fever, one must also consider the long-term hemodynamic effects of MS. The effect of MS on circulatory pressures and blood flow can

* Corresponding author. University of Colorado Health Sciences, 4200 East Ninth Avenue, Campus Box B132, University Hospital, Room 2017-B, Denver, CO 80262.

E-mail address: john.carroll@uchsc.edu (J.D. Carroll).

1551-7136/06/$ - see front matter © 2007 Elsevier Inc. All rights reserved.
doi:10.1016/j.hfc.2006.09.006

heartfailure.theclinics.com

be summarized in four separate and distinct clinical mechanisms: (1) increased transmitral pressure gradient in diastole, (2) increased transmitral blood velocity, (3) reduction in total flow across the valve, and (4) left atrial hypertension leading to increased pulmonary pressures and subsequent right ventricular overload [14]. These effects may contribute independently or in summation to the development of LV dysfunction in some patients.

Leading theories of etiologies of left ventricular dysfunction

MS inherently reflects a mechanical obstruction to flow from the left atrium to the left ventricle. For many years, this mechanical obstruction was believed to be the leading etiology of reduced cardiac function in patients who had MS (Table 1). Baker and colleagues [15,16] emphasized this effect as they explored the success of commissurotomy with the first reports of this treatment. The basis of this belief stemmed from the relief of symptoms after surgical intervention as the determination of LV function was limited at the time. With advances in technology, including the advent of indicator-dilution volumetric techniques and angiography, investigators began to quantitate MS-associated impaired LV dysfunction. Using dye-dilution techniques, Levinson and colleagues [17] were the first to demonstrate a reduced end-diastolic volume, reduced ejection fraction, and a significant decrease in cardiac output in 12 patients who had MS. This mechanical obstruction hypothesis was the leading theory of

Table 1
Proposed etiologies of the left ventricular dysfunction in mitral stenosis

---

1. Reduced filling of LV from mechanical obstruction from stenotic mitral valve
2. Chronic inflammation leading to abnormal wall motion from myocardial endofibrosis
3. Scarring of the subvalvular apparatus leading to wall motion abnormalities
4. Reduced LV compliance leading to profound diastolic function
5. Increased afterload leading to remodeling
6. Abnormal right-left septal interaction from pulmonary hypertension
7. Concomitant diseases such as systemic hypertension and coronary artery disease

---

clinical symptoms and of LV dysfunction into the 1950s [18].

In the 1950s, researchers began to raise the possibility that there may exist a factor specific to the left ventricle because some patients did not have relief of symptoms after surgical intervention. One of the initial proposed etiologies of LV dysfunction in MS was the effect of regional wall motion abnormalities. This theory developed with the advent of left heart catheterization, which permitted visual inspection of the LV cavity and assessment of motion by way of ventriculography. Holzer and colleagues [19] were among the first to attempt to angiographically quantify contraction abnormalities. In their study, they noted wall motion abnormalities in the basilar regions and suggested that this dysfunction could be residual from the initial rheumatic fever event [10]. Curry and colleagues [20] furthered this theory, noting additional wall motion abnormalities in the anterolateral wall of some patients who had MS. Abnormalities of the posterobasal and anterolateral walls were also found by Horwitz and colleagues [21] and Bolen and coworkers [22]. Hildner and colleagues [23] further qualitatively analyzed patients who had pure MS and reported LV enlargement and abnormal contraction in over half of their study population. This work spurred the search for the elusive myocardial factor because this was believed to be the cause of the reduced ejection and wall motion abnormalities present in these patients.

Grant [24] and then later Heller and Carleton [4] proposed an alternative theory for these wall motion abnormalities observed on ventriculography. Drawing from pathologic data first published in 1929 by Kirch [25], these investigators postulated that immobilization and atrophy of the posterobasilar wall might be related to thickening of the mitral apparatus, causing tethering and restriction of the adjacent myocardium with resultant segmental or regional dysfunction [10]. This implication of a malformed posterobasal area of the left ventricle as the probable origin of LV dysfunction was more evidence pointing to a myocardial versus a valvular etiology of LV dysfunction. This theory was further supported by work by Sunamori and colleagues [26] who found fibrosis in the myocardium at the base of papillary muscles removed at the time of mitral valve replacement (MVR).

From the concept of a restricted ventricle, either from tethering or from residual myocardial inflammation, the precept of reduced compliance arose. Feigenbaum and coworkers [27] first attempted to assess mean compliance using the ratio of mean mitral valve flow to change in chamber pressure versus time. Of interest, there was no difference in this study between control patients and MS patients. Since this initial study, many others have affirmed that the combination of a rigid mitral apparatus [4,20], chamber atrophy [24], potential endomyocardial fibrosis [28], and a contribution from the right-sided loading of the heart [20] leads to reduced compliance.

To investigate the potential effect of each factor upon compliance in isolation, Liu and colleagues [7] conducted an elegant study using conductance catheter/micromanometer techniques coupled with transient inferior vena cava (IVC) occlusion to alter loading conditions. In their study, the investigators compared nine patients with MS with eight age-matched controls. In a subset of the MS patients, measurements were obtained acutely and within 3 months after percutaneous mitral balloon valvuloplasty. These investigators noted several conclusions. First, they noted that the finding of reduced diastolic compliance was reversed shortly after valvuloplasty. As endomyocardial fibrosis should not be acutely reversed by any procedure, these investigators rejected this hypothesis. Second, the theory of chamber atrophy from chronic underfilling was also refuted on the immediate effect of valvuloplasty on the pressure volume curves. Third, by measuring the end-diastolic pressure volume curves with complete unloading of the right ventricle by way of IVC occlusion, they rejected the effect of the right ventricle upon diastolic compliance. In addition, after balloon valvuloplasty, there was a substantial increase in left ventricular chamber compliance that essentially equaled that of the right ventricle. The conclusion of the study was that the etiology of reduced diastolic compliance seen in MS must be the immobility of the mitral apparatus. Liu and colleagues [7] likened this tethering effect to pericardial constriction and percutaneous mitral balloon valvotomy (PMBV) to release of this constriction by sheering of the mechanical constraint and subsequent return to normal diastolic function.

One precept of the mechanical obstruction hypothesis was that the pure underfilling of the left ventricle contributed to its impaired performance. Many investigators explored the relationship between LV end-diastolic volumes and impaired LV dysfunction. The results have been conflicting, with some investigators reporting smaller than normal LV end-diastolic volumes [6,20] and others noting normal or increased volumes [5,29–31]. Wisenbaugh and colleagues [32] reported similar end-diastolic volumes, end-diastolic pressures, and end-diastolic wall stress among patients who had MS and an ejection fraction less than 55%, patients who had MS and an ejection fraction greater than 55%, and control patients. McKay and coworkers [33] measured preload before and after percutaneous valvuloplasty and showed that end-diastolic volumes did not increase at all or increased very little after the procedure. Furthermore, Wisenbaugh and the procedure [32] noted a modest increase in preload measurements after valvuloplasty in patients who had MS and reduced ejection fraction (<55%), without normalization of ejection fraction. Therefore, most agree that the underfilling hypothesis has been successfully refuted as an etiology of impaired LV dysfunction in pure MS.

Increased afterload has been examined also as a potential cause of LV dysfunction in MS. Gash and colleagues [6] proposed that the reduction in ejection fraction can be explained by high afterload that is not met by an increase in preload due to the reduction in mitral valve orifice seen in MS. They hypothesized that the higher afterload is a result of inadequate end-systolic wall thickness, which in turn increases wall stress at a normal LV systolic pressure. Kaku and colleagues [31] and Mohan and coworkers [5] independently found similar evidence for increased afterload in this patient population. Wisenbaugh and colleagues [32] investigated the effect of valvuloplasty on afterload, noting no significant decrease despite an apparent increase in preload. The conclusion from this study proposed that there was yet another unmeasured factor, perhaps endothelin, that results in higher peripheral vascular resistance and vasoconstriction in this patient population [29,32].

Further evidence for an altered neurohormonal axis can be demonstrated in patients who have MS. Ashino and colleagues [34] demonstrated neurohormonal activation by showing increased serum concentrations of various neurotransmitters and their metabolites and by examining microneurographically measured muscle sympathetic nerve activity. The stimulus for this activation is thought to be altered hemodynamics given that this increased sympathetic activity in MS is completely reversed 1 week after PMBV [1]. The well-known alterations in the renin-angiotensin-aldosterone system seen in other etiologies of heart

failure have not been fully explored in this patient population. This deficit is likely due to
the recent ability to assess these changes in the
setting of a decreasing patient population that
has MS and LV dysfunction.

Long-standing MS is a well-known cause of
pulmonary hypertension, which in turn can affect
right ventricular function. An association often
cited has been the presence of an impaired right
ventricle with an impaired left ventricle. In many
patients who have MS, a brief posterior or
leftward motion of the interventricular septum is
prominent in early diastole, just after the mitral
valve opens [10]. The exaggerated displacement of
the septum is due to unequal filling of the two ventricles [10,35]. Given the mechanical obstruction
to LV filling and the lack of obstruction on the
right side, early diastolic filling is more rapid in
the right ventricle versus the left ventricle. This
rapid inflow coupled with the diastolic suction
component from the left side results in the leftward movement of the interventricular septum
seen in MS. The effects on the septum from the
pulmonary hypertension induced by MS have
been implicated in impaired LV function. In
fact, the septum may be hypertrophied, hypoki-
netic, or dyskinetic [36–38]. These septal abnormalities, per some investigators, may contribute
to the decrease in LV systolic function seen in
some patients with MS.

MS provides a milieu for diastolic dysfunction,
which is a common cause of heart failure. In the
presence of LV diastolic dysfunction, the symptoms of dyspnea and the degree of increase in left
atrial pressure may be more than expected from
the severity of the MS [1]. The deleterious effect of
diastolic dysfunction in patients who have MS
was shown by studies performed by Sabbah and
colleagues [39] and Paulus and coworkers [40].
These investigators, by way of micromanometer
recordings, demonstrated that negative intraventricular pressures are generated in early diastole
in patients who have MS (Fig. 1). This diastolic
suction effect provides less reliance on atrial contraction for LV filling. When diastolic dysfunction
ensues, most commonly from hypertensive heart
disease, this mechanism of filling is lost. In addition, one may see an increase in late diastolic pressure in these patients due to the concomitant
presence of diastolic dysfunction. The combination of these two deleterious effects can contribute
to a profound increase in symptoms. Hence, both
systolic and diastolic function are important in
patients who have MS.

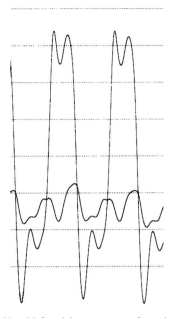

Fig. 1. LV and left atrial pressure waveforms in MS. Although these recordings were made with fluid-filled systems, micromanometer recordings have shown that LV
pressure can be negative in early diastole in patients
who have MS. The generation of negative pressure is
due to the normal generation of a suction force in the
left ventricle during early diastole accompanied by restricted inflow due to the MS. The end-diastolic pressure
is elevated in this example. In the individual patient, the
causes for the elevated LV end-diastolic pressure are variable but may include reduced chamber compliance due
to the tethering effect of the mitral apparatus in MS.

In addition to hypertensive heart disease,
coronary artery disease (CAD) is another common cause of impaired LV systolic and diastolic
function in this patient population. The frequency
of coronary disease in this patient population
varies depending on which age group is surveyed.
Mattina and colleagues [41] attempted to assess
the prevalence of CAD in patients who had MS
and the reliability of the symptoms of angina pectoris to predict coronary disease. In their retrospective study of 96 patients, they found
angiographically significant coronary disease in
27 (28%) of their population. These patients
were all over age 40 years. In addition, they determined that the presence of angina had a sensitivity
of 37% and a specificity of 84% for CAD. They
concluded that CAD in patients with MS who
are older than 40 years of age is common and often clinically silent. In contrast, a more recent
study by Guray and colleagues [42] noted

a different threshold for coronary angiography. In their study of 837 patients (35–77 years old), they found a prevalence of only 7.5% of angiographically significant (defined as greater than 50% narrowing) CAD. They noted that the presence of angina pectoris had a sensitivity of 33.3%, a specificity of 86.3%, a positive predictive value of 16.5%, and a negative predictive value of 94.1%. Guray and colleagues [42] concluded that routine coronary angiography is not necessarily indicated in patients with MS, particularly in patients who are younger than 40 years of age and have no coronary risk factors or angina pectoris. Overall, the prevalence of coronary disease without traditional risk factors is thought to be low in this population. Therefore, angiography to determine the cause of LV dysfunction in patients who have MS should likely be limited to patients who have traditional CAD risk factors.

Diagnosis of left ventricular dysfunction in mitral stenosis

Echocardiography and the determination of ejection fraction is the main current method to diagnose LV dysfunction in MS (Fig. 2). Although ejection fractions derived from echocardiography are often used to drive clinical practice, they tend to be subjective and variable [43]. Much of this is due to the load-dependent variables measured and the high prevalence of atrial

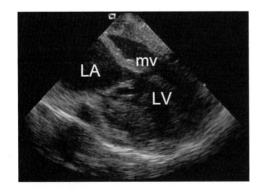

Fig. 2. An intracardiac ultrasound from a patient who had MS. Note the thickening of the anterior leaflet, the small chamber size, and the normal LV wall thickness. During systole, there was normal chamber contraction and normal wall thickening. Often, LV systolic function is normal and, even when the ejection fraction is somewhat reduced in MS, it does not appear to impact on surgical mortality. LA, left atrium; MV, mitral valve.

fibrillation seen in this patient population. This subjectivity has undoubtedly led to the varying rates reported of LV dysfunction with MS. With the development of Doppler tissue imaging (DTI) and strain rate imaging (SRI), recent studies have begun to report indices of subclinical LV dysfunction in this patient population that are not load dependent. Ozer and colleagues [44], on the basis that LV long-axis function evaluated by M-mode or tissue Doppler echocardiography is a practical index of LV function [45,46], reported that these indices are reduced in patients who have MS. Of interest, these investigators explored these markers of LV function in patients who were thought to have normal LV ejection fraction as assessed by fractional shortening. Similarly, using DTI, Ozdemir and colleagues [47] showed that in patients who have pure MS, there was a reduction in LV systolic and diastolic myocardial velocities. Thus, these investigators demonstrated LV dysfunction in patients who had proposed normal ejection fractions by standard echocardiography.

Working on the basis that DTI can be difficult to use clinically, Dogan and coworkers [48] proposed another method to assess LV function in MS patients, namely, strain rate and strain rate imaging (SRI). This new technique, which is derived from DTI, allows the determination of velocity gradients between two myocardial points [49]. One attractive aspect of using this method is that SRI is not affected by the rotation and translation of the whole heart, contraction of adjacent segments, or basoapical velocity gradients that complicate segmental analysis of diastolic function [48,50]. Dogan and coworkers [48] showed that there was impaired long-axis function in patients who had mild to moderate MS and normal global systolic function. This recent study is of interest in its use of strain rate and SRI. The determination of global long-axis function by way of these methods was recently shown to be able to predict contractile reserve in asymptomatic patients who had severe mitral regurgitation [51]. If the use of these new techniques is widely adopted, then the prevalence of LV dysfunction in MS may dramatically rise.

The use of serum markers, specifically B-type natriuretic peptide (BNP), has become commonplace in the diagnosis of patients who have heart failure. It is unfortunate that little information exists regarding the use of BNP in patients who have valvular heart disease. The use of BNP in patients who have MS remains controversial. In various studies, BNP levels have clearly been shown to be elevated in patients who have MS [52,53]; however, there has been a lack of correlation between the severity of MS and BNP levels. Yoshimura and colleagues [52] found higher levels of BNP in patients who had MS compared with controls, but also found no correlation with level of BNP and wedge pressure. Most recently, two separate studies [54,55] have investigated the precursor to BNP (ie, N-terminal [NT]-proBNP). Both studies reported that NT-proBNP correlates positively with MS severity. In addition, Arat-Ozkan and colleagues [54] correlated NT pro-BNP with functional class and proposed this method as a manner to follow patients who have MS. It is unfortunate that although NT-proBNP correlated well with left atrial and right ventricular dimensions, New York Heart Association (NYHA) class, and mitral valve area, there was no investigation as per the use of NT-proBNP in patients who had MS and a reduced ejection fraction. Although there have been recent data on the use of BNP as a useful clinical marker in determining optimal surgical timing in valvular heart disease patients [56], data investigating or guiding the use of BNP in patients who have MS and LV dysfunction are nonexistent.

Other serum markers can also be elevated in rheumatic MS, including C-reactive protein [57], circulating adhesion molecules [58], and even tumor markers such as CA-125 [59]. The only marker that has been correlated with heart failure has been CA-125. This finding echoes other reports of increased tumor markers occasionally seen in heart failure patients. The proposed mechanism is venous congestion and subsequent activation of the peritoneal mesothelium. Although interesting, there have been no studies demonstrating a clear biomarker that will successfully predict the presence of LV dysfunction in MS.

Treatment of left ventricular dysfunction in mitral stenosis

Mitral valve replacement

Mitral valve replacement (MVR) is currently recommended (Class I) for patients who have moderate to severe MS with NYHA class III or IV symptoms who are not considered candidates for mitral balloon valvulotomy [60]. It is a class IIa indication in for patients who have NYHA class I and II symptoms with severe pulmonary hypertension who are not candidates for balloon valvulotomy. With respect to ejection fraction,

no studies have provided clear evidence of improved ejection performance after surgical therapy for MS [61–63].

Little data exists regarding the outcomes in patients who have reduced ejection fraction with MVR. Snyder and colleagues [8] investigated the influence of preoperative ejection fraction in an MS population undergoing surgical commissurotomy or MVR. In their study, they found that preoperative ejection fraction did not predict perioperative mortality or short-term symptomatic response.

The issue of preservation of chordae with MVR was addressed by Chowdhury and colleagues [64]. They reviewed patients who had rheumatic MS and underwent MVR with complete excision of subvalvular apparatus, preservation of the posterior chordopapillary apparatus, or total chordal preservation (Fig. 3). Total or posterior chordopapillary preservation was associated with lower incidence of low cardiac output and better long-term survival. In the group with complete chordal excision, the LV ejection fraction was significantly decreased postoperatively and continued to decline over time and did not improve by 4 years. It is unfortunate that the patient population in this study was tainted by mixed mitral valve disease, which limits the extraction of this study given the known benefit of chordal preservation in patients who have mitral regurgitation. In addition, this study did not strictly include patients who had a reduced

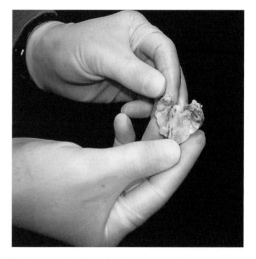

Fig. 3. A surgically excised mitral valve in a patient who has MS demonstrates the fibrosis and thickening of a leaflet and a portion of the subvalvular apparatus.

ejection fraction, which further limits the generalizability of this data.

The best study that addressed patients who had a reduced ejection fraction and MS undergoing MVR was performed by Mangoni and coworkers [65]. These investigators evaluated 16 patients who had MS without significant mitral regurgitation with an LV ejection fraction less than 50% (mean, 0.45) and compared them with patients who had MS and an ejection fraction greater than 60% (mean, 0.66). All patients underwent MVR and were followed closely for morbidity and mortality. In patients who had a reduced ejection fraction, there was a higher incidence of in-hospital heart failure and an increase in heart failure–related deaths. There was no difference, however, in overall mortality, rate of cardiac admission, or mean Specific Activity Scale score. The investigators concluded that moderate depression of LV ejection fraction should not be a contraindication to MVR for MS.

Percutaneous mitral balloon valvotomy

PMBV has provided an arena in which to study the effect of relieving the ventricular inflow obstruction inherent to this disease. Given that one leading theory of reduced LV function is impaired inflow, PMBV should affect LV ejection fraction by removal of the obstruction. It is unfortunate that this has been yet another topic of debate.

Although there have been no studies strictly including patients who have LV dysfunction, there have been numerous reports on the effects of PMBV on LV end-diastolic volume, LV end-diastolic pressure, and ejection fraction. Several studies have demonstrated that PMBV improves diastolic filling and increases end-diastolic volume immediately [66–69]. Other investigators have shown the contrary, with no response in these indices with PMBV [32,70–72]. In the studies with an improvement in filling indices, the ejection fraction was also shown to increase [66,67,69]. To complicate the matter further, in the studies by Fawzy and colleagues [66] and Yasuda and colleagues [69], LV end-diastolic volumes and ejection fraction continued to improve at follow-up after PMBV. Fawzy and colleagues [66] also noted an increased systemic vascular resistance at baseline, corroborating the theory of increased afterload in these patients. Most important, this increased peripheral resistance was noted to be markedly decreased when measured 12 months after PMBV. Although no studies have specifically addressed patients who have reduced ejection fraction, extrapolation from the aforementioned studies suggests a neutral or a positive effect of PMBV on indices of LV function.

Medical therapy

There are limited data regarding the medical therapy of patients who have MS and LV dysfunction. Although β-blockade is common in patients who have MS, valvular heart disease is often an exclusion criterion for heart failure trials, leading to a large void in the optimal treatment of these patients. Angiotensin-converting enzyme (ACE) inhibition has been classically seen as contraindicated given the fear of hypotension in the setting of a fixed obstruction. Sebastian and colleagues [73] investigated the effect of ACE inhibition in three patients who had severe MS in whom surgery was delayed. These investigators reported an initial improvement in symptoms and, more important, ACE inhibition did not cause an excessive fall in blood pressure or impairment of renal function. The largest trial to date using ACE inhibitors in patients who had MS came from Chockalingam and coworkers [74] who studied 109 patients who had MS and NYHA class III and IV symptoms. The patient population in this study included mixed mitral valve disease and some patients concomitant aortic valve disease. The findings were that irrespective of valve pathology, the use of an ACE inhibitor (enalapril) improved functional status and exercise capacity. It was not surprising that the greatest effects were in patients who had concomitant regurgitant valvular heart disease. It is unfortunate that no measure of ejection fraction was made for this study, but extrapolation from thousands of patients in heart failure studies suggests that patients who have MS and reduced ejection fraction would also benefit from ACE inhibition. At the current time, however, no specific data for this population exist as per the optimal medical regimen.

Summary

A reduced ejection fraction in the setting of MS is relatively commonplace, with a prevalence of approximately 30%. The etiologies of the impairment have been attributed to impaired diastolic filling, impaired myocardial contractility, excessive LV afterload, rigidity and fixation of the posterobasal LV myocardium from scarring or concomitant inflammation, effects from the right ventricle, or a combination of these forces [65]. Although there is much debate, most likely the etiology of impaired LV function in patients with MS is patient specific and multifactorial in nature. The diagnosis of impaired LV function can be difficult with current methodologies given the subjectivity and load dependence of echocardiography, although new methods are being developed. The treatment of MS with LV dysfunction appears to be moot, in that all invasive treatments except those involving chordal excision appear to be beneficial. Medical therapy of these conditions is currently limited. Although standard of care involves β-blockade for prolongation of diastolic filling time, which also provides benefit in LV dysfunction, there are some data regarding ACE inhibition. Regardless, a reduced ejection fraction does not appear to alter long-term outcomes, either surgical or percutaneous.

References

[1] Carroll JD, Sutherland JP, Mitral stenosis in cardiology. 2nd edition. In: Crawford MH, DiMarco JP, Paulus WJ, et al, editors. London: Mosby Int; 2003.

[2] Waller BF, Howard J, Fess S. Pathology of mitral valve stenosis and pure mitral regurgitation—part II. Clin Cardiol 1994;17:395–402.

[3] Carabello BA. Modern management of mitral stenosis. Circulation 2005;112:432–7.

[4] Heller SJ, Carleton RA. Abnormal left ventricular contraction in patients with mitral stenosis. Circulation 1970;42:1099–119.

[5] Mohan JC, Khalilullah M, Arora R. Left ventricular intrinsic contractility in pure rheumatic mitral stenosis. Am J Cardiol 1989;64:240–2.

[6] Gash AK, Carabello BA, Cepini D, et al. Left ventricular ejection performance and systolic muscle function in patients with mitral stenosis. Circulation 1983;67(1):148–54.

[7] Liu CP, Ting CT, Yang TM, et al. Reduced left ventricular compliance in human mitral stenosis. Role of reversible internal constraint. Circulation 1992; 85:1447–56.

[8] Snyder RW II, Lange RA, Willard JE, et al. Frequency, cause and effect on operative outcome of depressed left ventricular ejection fraction in mitral stenosis. Am J Cardiol 1994;73(1):65–9.

[9] Choi BW, Bacharach SL, Barbour DJ, et al. Left ventricular systolic dysfunction diastolic filling characteristics and exercise cardiac reserve in mitral stenosis. Am J Cardiol 1995;75(7):526–9.

[10] Gaasch WH, Folland D. Left ventricular function in rheumatic mitral stenosis. Eur Heart J 1991; 12(Suppl B):66–9.

[11] Harvey RM, Ferrer MI, Samet P, et al. Mechanical and myocardial factors in rheumatic heart disease with mitral stenosis. Circulation 1955;11:531–51.

[12] Fleming HA, Woop P. The myocardial factor in mitral valve disease. Br Heart J 1959;21:117–22.

[13] Waller BF, Howard J, Fess S. Pathology of mitral valve stenosis and pure mitral regurgitation—part I. Clin Cardiol 1994;17:330–6.

[14] Abbo KM, Carroll JD. Hemodynamics of mitral stenosis: a review. Cathet Cardiovasc Diag 1994;2: 16–25.

[15] Baker C, Brock RC, Campbell M. Valvulotomy for mitral stenosis: report of six successful cases. Br Med J 1950;4665:1283–93.

[16] Baker C, Brock RC, Campbell M, et al. Valvulotomy for mitral stenosis: a further report, on 100 cases. Br Med J 1952;4767:1043–55.

[17] Levinson GE, Frank MJ, Nadimi M, et al. Studies of cardiopulmonary blood volume. Measurement of left ventricular volume by dye dilution. Circulation 1967;35(6):1038–48.

[18] Hugenholtz PG, Ryan TJ, Stein SW, et al. The spectrum of pure mitral stenosis. Hemodynamic studies in relation to clinical disability. Am J Cardiol 1962; 10:773–84.

[19] Holzer JA, Karliner JS, O'Rourke RA, et al. Quantitative angiographic analysis of the left ventricle in patients with isolated rheumatic mitral stenosis. Br Heart J 1973;35:497–502.

[20] Curry GC, Elliott LP, Ramsey HW. Quantitative left ventricular angiographic finding in mitral stenosis. Am J Cardiol 1972;29:621–7.

[21] Horwitz LD, Mullins CB, Payne PM, et al. Left ventricular function in mitral stenosis. Chest 1973;64: 609–14.

[22] Bolen JL, Lopes MG, Harrison DC, et al. Analysis of left ventricular function in response to afterload changes in patients with mitral stenosis. Circulation 1975;52:894.

[23] Hildner FJ, Javier RP, Cohen LS, et al. Myocardial dysfunction associated with valvular heart diseases. Am J Cardiol 1972;30:319–26.

[24] Grant RP. Architectonics of the heart. Am Heart J 1953;46:405–31.

[25] Kirch E. Alterations in size and shape of individual regions of the heart in valvular heart disease. Verh Deutsch Ges Inn Med Kong 1929;41: 324–31.

[26] Sunamori M, Suzuki A, Harrison CE. Relationship between left ventricular morphology and postoperative cardiac function following valve replacement for mitral stenosis. J Thorac Cardiovasc Surg 1983; 85(5):727–32.

[27] Feigenbaum H, Campbell RW, Wunsch CM, et al. Evaluation of the left ventricle in patients with mitral stenosis. Circulation 1966;34:462–72.

[28] Grismer JT, Anderson WR, Weiss L. Chronic occlusive rheumatic coronary vasculitis and myocardial dysfunction. Am J Cardiol 1967;20:739–45.

[29] Ahmed SS, Regan TJ, Fiore JJ, et al. The state of the left ventricular myocardium in mitral stenosis. Am Heart J 1977;94:28–36.

[30] Daoud ZF. Left ventricular function in isolated mitral stenosis: echocardiographic assessment. Curr Ther Res 1985;37:607–13.

[31] Kaku K, Hirota Y, Shimizu G, et al. Depressed myocardial contractility in mitral stenosis—an analysis by force-length and stress-shortening relationships. Jpn Circ J 1988;52:35–43.

[32] Wisenbaugh T, Essop R, Middlemost S, et al. Excessive vasoconstriction in rheumatic mitral stenosis with modestly reduced ejection fraction. J Am Coll Cardiol 1992;20:1339–44.

[33] McKay CR, Kawanishi DT, Kotlewski A, et al. Improvement in exercise capacity and exercise hemodynamics 3 months after double-balloon, catheter balloon valvuloplasty treatment of patients with symptomatic mitral stenosis. Circulation 1988; 77(5):1013–21.

[34] Ashino K, Gotoh E, Sumita S, et al. Percutaneous transluminal mitral valvuloplasty normalizes baroreflex sensitivity and sympathetic activity in patients with mitral stenosis. Circulation 1997;96(10): 3443–9.

[35] Weyman AE, Heger JJ, Kronik G, et al. Mechanism of paradoxical early diastolic septal motion in patients with mitral stenosis: a cross-sectional echocardiographic study. Am J Cardiol 1977;40: 691–9.

[36] Kelly DT, Spotnitz HM, Beiser GD, et al. Effects of chronic right ventricular volume and pressure loading on left ventricular performance. Circulation 1971;44(3):403–12.

[37] Bemis CE, Serur JR, Borkenhagen D, et al. Influence of right ventricular filling pressure on left ventricular pressure and dimension. Circ Res 1974;34(4): 498–504.

[38] Akaishi M, Akizuki S, Nanda S, et al. Left ventricular shape and function in patients with chronic right ventricular overloading. J Cardiogr 1980;10:153–61.

[39] Sabbah HN, Anbe DT, Stein PD. Negative intraventricular diastolic pressure in patients with mitral stenosis: evidence of left ventricular diastolic suction. Am J Cardiol 1980;45:562–6.

[40] Paulus WJ, Vantrimpont PJ, Rousseau MF. Diastolic function of the nonfilling human left ventricle. J Am Coll Cardiol 1992;20:1524–32.

[41] Mattina CJ, Green SJ, Tortolani AJ, et al. Frequency of angiographically significant coronary arterial narrowing in mitral stenosis. Am J Cardiol 1986;57(10):802–5.

[42] Guray Y, Guray U, Yilmaz MB, et al. Prevalence of angiographically significant coronary artery disease in patients with rheumatic mitral stenosis. Acta Cardiol 2004;59(3):305–9.

[43] Kuecherer HF, Kee LL, Modin G, et al. Echocardiography in serial evaluation of left ventricular systolic and diastolic function: importance of image acquisition, quantitation, and physiologic variability in clinical and investigational applications. J Am Soc Echocardiogr 1991;4(3):203–14.

[44] Ozer N, Can I, Atalar E, et al. Left ventricular long-axis function is reduced in patients with rheumatic mitral stenosis. Echocardiography 2004;21(2): 107–12.

[45] Simonson JS, Schiller NB. Descent of the base of the left ventricle: an echocardiographic index of left ventricular function. J Am Soc Echo 1989;2:25–35.

[46] Gulati VK, Katz WE, Follansbee WP, et al. Mitral annular descent velocity by tissue Doppler echocardiography as an index of global left ventricular function. Am J Cardiol 1996;77(11):979–84.

[47] Ozdemir K, Altunkeser BB, Gok H, et al. Analysis of the myocardial velocities in patients with mitral stenosis. J Am Soc Echocardiogr 2002;15(12): 1472–8.

[48] Dogan S, Aydin M, Gursurer M, et al. Prediction of subclinical left ventricular dysfunction with strain rate imaging in patients with mild to moderate rheumatic mitral stenosis. J Am Soc Echocardiogr 2006; 19(3):243–8.

[49] Heimdal A, Stoylen A, Torp H, et al. Real-time strain rate imaging of the left ventricle by ultrasound. J Am Soc Echocardiogr 1998;11(11):1013–9.

[50] D'hooge J, Heimdal A, Jamal F, et al. Regional strain and strain rate measurements by cardiac ultrasound: principles, implementation and limitations. Eur J Echocardiogr 2000;1(3):154–70.

[51] Lee R, Hanekom L, Marwick TH, et al. Prediction of subclinical left ventricular dysfunction with strain rate imaging in patients with asymptomatic severe mitral regurgitation. Am J Cardiol 2004;94(10): 1333–7.

[52] Yoshimura M, Yasue H, Okumura K, et al. Different secretion patterns of atrial natriuretic peptide and brain natriuretic peptide in patients with congestive heart failure. Circulation 1993;87(2): 464–9.

[53] Nakamura M, Kawata Y, Yoshida H, et al. Relationship between plasma atrial and brain natriuretic peptide concentration and hemodynamic parameters during percutaneous transvenous mitral valvulotomy in patients with mitral stenosis. Am Heart J 1992;124(5):1283–8.

[54] Arat-Ozkan A, Kaya A, Yigit Z, et al. Serum N-terminal pro-BNP levels correlate with symptoms and echocardiographic findings in patients with mitral stenosis. Echocardiography 2005;22(6):473–8.

[55] Iltumur K, Karabulut A, Yokus B, et al. N-terminal proBNP plasma levels correlate with severity of mitral stenosis. J Heart Valve Dis 2005;14(6):735–41.

[56] Watanabe M, Murakami M, Furukawa H, et al. Is measurement of plasma brain natriuretic peptide levels a useful test to detect for surgical timing of valve disease? Int J Cardiol 2004;96(1):21–4.

[57] Krasuski RA, Bush A, Kay JE, et al. C-reactive protein elevation independently influences the

procedural success of percutaneous balloon mitral valve commissurotomy. Am Heart J 2003;146(6): 1099–104.

[58] Yetkin E, Erbay AR, Turhan H, et al. Changes in plasma levels of adhesion molecules after percutaneous mitral balloon valvuloplasty. Cardiovasc Pathol 2004;13(2):103–8.

[59] Duman C, Ercan E, Tengiz I, et al. Elevated serum CA 125 levels in mitral stenotic patients with heart failure. Cardiology 2003;100(1):7–10.

[60] Bonow RO, Carabello B, Kanu C, et al. ACC/AHA 2006 guidelines for the management of patients with valvular heart disease: a report of the American College of Cardiology/American Heart Association Task Force on Practice Guidelines (writing committee to revise the 1998 Guidelines for the Management of Patients with Valvular Heart Disease)—developed in collaboration with the Society of Cardiovascular Anesthesiologists, endorsed by the Society for Cardiovascular Angiography and Interventions and the Society of Thoracic Surgeons. Circulation 2006;114(5):e84–231.

[61] Kennedy JW, Doces JG, Stewart DK. Left ventricular function before and following surgical treatment of mitral valve disease. Am Heart J 1979;97(5):592–8.

[62] Johnston DL, Lesoway R, Kostuk WJ. Ventricular function following mitral valve surgery: assessment using radionuclide ventriculography. Can J Surg 1984;27(4):349–53.

[63] Kazama S, Nishiguchi K, Sonoda K, et al. Postoperative left ventricular function in patients with mitral stenosis. The effect of commissurotomy and valve replacement on left ventricular systolic function. Jpn Heart J 1986;27(1):35–42.

[64] Chowdhury UK, Kumar AS, Airan B, et al. Mitral valve replacement with and without chordal preservation in a rheumatic population: serial echocardiographic assessment of left ventricular size and function. Ann Thorac Surg 2005;79(6):1926–33.

[65] Mangoni AA, Koelling TM, Meyer GS, et al. Outcome following mitral valve replacement in patients with mitral stenosis and moderately reduced left ventricular ejection fraction. Eur J Cardiothorac Surg 2002;22(1):90–4.

[66] Fawzy ME, Choi WB, Mimish L, et al. Immediate and long-term effect of mitral balloon valvotomy on left ventricular volume and systolic function in severe mitral stenosis. Am Heart J 1996;132(2 Pt 1): 356–60.

[67] Goto S, Handa S, Akaishi M, et al. Left ventricular ejection performance in mitral stenosis, and effects of successful percutaneous transvenous mitral commissurotomy. Am J Cardiol 1992;69(3):233–7.

[68] Tischler MD, Sutton MS, Bittl JA, et al. Effects of percutaneous mitral valvuloplasty on left ventricular mass and volume. Am J Cardiol 1991;68(9):940–4.

[69] Yasuda S, Nagata S, Tamai J, et al. Left ventricular diastolic pressure-volume response immediately after successful percutaneous transvenous mitral commissurotomy. Am J Cardiol 1993;71(11):932–7.

[70] Harrison JK, Davidson CJ, Hermiller JB, et al. Left ventricular filling and ventricular diastolic performance after percutaneous balloon mitral valvotomy. Am J Cardiol 1992;69(1):108–12.

[71] Mohan JC, Nair M, Arora R. Left ventricular volumes and function immediately after balloon mitral valvoplasty. Int J Cardiol 1991;33(2):275–80.

[72] Pamir G, Ertas F, Oral D, et al. Left ventricular filling and ejection fraction after successful percutaneous balloon mitral valvuloplasty. Int J Cardiol 1997;59(3):243–6.

[73] Sebastian VJ, Bhattacharya S, Ray S, et al. Beneficial effects of ACE inhibitors in severe mitral stenosis. Med J Malaysia 1989;44(4):291–5.

[74] Chockalingam A, Venkatesan S, Dorairajan S, et al. Safety and efficacy of enalapril in multivalvular heart disease with significant mitral stenosis— SCOPE-MS. Angiology 2005;56(2):151–8.

ELSEVIER
SAUNDERS

Heart Failure Clin 2 (2006) 453–460

**HEART
FAILURE
CLINICS**

Hemodynamic Characteristics and Progression to Heart Failure in Regurgitant Lesions

Vera H. Rigolin, MD*, Robert O. Bonow, MD

Feinberg School of Medicine, Northwestern University, Chicago, IL, USA

Mitral and aortic valvular regurgitation are two lesions that share the common denominator of left ventricular (LV) volume overload. Both lesions, in severe cases, can result in progressive LV dilatation, systolic dysfunction, and clinical heart failure in the absence of correction. Despite these similarities, the pathophysiology of LV adaptation to the volume-overload states created by mitral regurgitation (MR) and aortic regurgitation (AR) is distinctly different, as are the clinical sequelae and outcomes. This article reviews the mechanisms of disease, compensation, and eventual decompensation in both disorders.

Mitral regurgitation

MR can be a primary disorder when the structure of the mitral valve is altered. These intrinsic components of the mitral valve apparatus include the leaflets, the annulus, the chordea tendinae, and the papillary muscles [1]. MR can also develop as a secondary process due to disorders of the myocardium that result in LV dilatation, regional systolic dysfunction annular dilatation, altered papillary muscle geometry, and tethering of the mitral valve leaflets [1–4]. In the United States, the most common cause of MR is mitral valve prolapse, whereas ischemic MR is second leading cause [2]. Identifying the cause of MR is crucial for understanding the natural history of the disorder and for defining the appropriate treatment strategy.

* Corresponding author. Feinberg School of Medicine, Northwestern University, 201 E. Huron, Galter 10-240, Chicago, IL 60611.

E-mail address: v-rigolin@northwestern.edu (V.H. Rigolin).

Mechanisms of compensation for volume overload

MR sufficient to cause significant volume overload may progress through three different stages, as depicted in Fig. 1. In the acute stage, MR may be catastrophic due to the rapid increase in volume into left-sided chambers that have not yet been able to compensate. This scenario results in decreased forward cardiac output and subsequent left atrial and pulmonary venous hypertension. The increase in volume into the left ventricle stretches the LV sarcomeres, thus activating the Frank-Starling mechanism, resulting in modest increases in diastolic volume and stroke work. Regurgitation of blood into the left atrium results in a decrease in LV systolic volume. These two effects result in an increase in total LV stroke volume. Because a large percentage of blood is directed toward the left atrium, however, forward stroke volume is reduced, and tachycardia develops as a prerequisite to maintain forward cardiac output. The left atrium is ill prepared for the sudden increase in volume, resulting in pulmonary congestion [5]. Thus, tachycardia, pulmonary congestion, and hypotension (and even frank cardiogenic shock) are common aspects of acute MR.

When a patient survives the acute episode of MR or has slowly progressive mitral valve disease, chronic compensation occurs, often resulting in very few symptoms.

In this phase, the LV sarcomeres are added in series, increasing the overall length of individual cardiomyocytes. The resultant LV dilatation and eccentric hypertrophy cause an increase in LV end-diastolic volume. Afterload (wall stress) increases from subnormal to normal according to Laplace's law (wall stress = pressure × radius/ thickness × 2). The left atrium also enlarges, thus

1551-7136/06/$ - see front matter © 2007 Elsevier Inc. All rights reserved.
doi:10.1016/j.hfc.2006.09.009

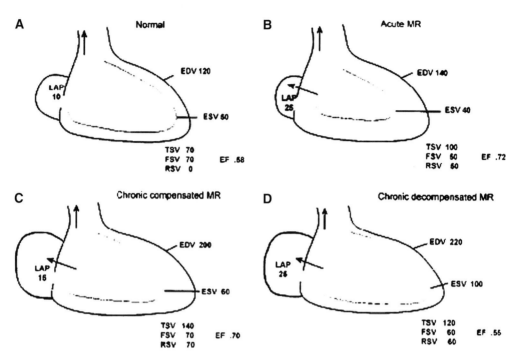

Fig. 1. The different phases of MR are displayed. (*A*) Normal physiology. EDV, end-diastolic volume; EF, ejection fraction; ESV, end-systolic volume; FSV, forward stroke volume; LAP, left atrial pressure; RSV, regurgitant stroke volume; TSV, total stroke volume. (*B*) Acute MR. Note the increased preload and decreased afterload. EDV is increased, ESV is decreased, and thus TSV is increased. Note that 50% of TSV is directed into the left atrium, thus increasing LAP. (*C*) Compensated phase. Here, eccentric hypertrophy has developed and EDV has increased substantially. Afterload has normalized. These compensatory mechanisms allow a significant increase in TSV compared with the acute phase. The enlarged left atrium can now accommodate a higher volume at a lower pressure. (*D*) Chronic decompensated phase. Muscle dysfunction has developed, resulting in a marked increase in ESV. EF, although still normal, has declined to 55%. LAP is increased due to the elevated EDV. (*From* Carabello BA. Mitral valve regurgitation. Curr Probl Cardiol 1998;23(4):205; with permission.)

allowing accommodation of the regurgitant volume at a lower pressure [5].

There is also a modest increase in LV mass that contributes to the compensatory process. Unlike aortic stenosis, however, in which compensation occurs by increased protein synthesis, patients who have MR compensate by reduced degradation [6,7]. Eccentric hypertrophy, enhanced preload, normal wall stress, and normal contractile function allow normal LV performance [2].

Patients who have compensated MR may remain in this phase for varying periods, often for decades. If the regurgitation is severe enough, however, decompensation may eventually result. The now-weakened left ventricle can no longer expel the excess volume, resulting in an increase in LV end-systolic volume. Forward stroke volume is again decreased and LV filling pressure and left atrial pressure are increased. Ejection fraction in all three phases, however, may be greater than

normal due to the increase in preload and the afterload-reducing effect of ejection into the low-impedance left atrium. Thus, ejection fraction can be misleading as a measure of compensation in this disorder, and advanced myocardial dysfunction may occur while LV ejection fraction is still well in the normal range [5].

Mechanisms of left ventricular dysfunction in chronic mitral regurgitation

The causes of LV decompensation at the cellular level in this disorder are multifactorial and highly complex. Studies in experimental models of MR in dogs and analysis of papillary muscles in patients who underwent surgical correction of MR demonstrate reduced myocin content and a loss of contractile elements (Fig. 2) [8–10]. A deficiency in cyclic AMP production resulting in altered excitation–contraction

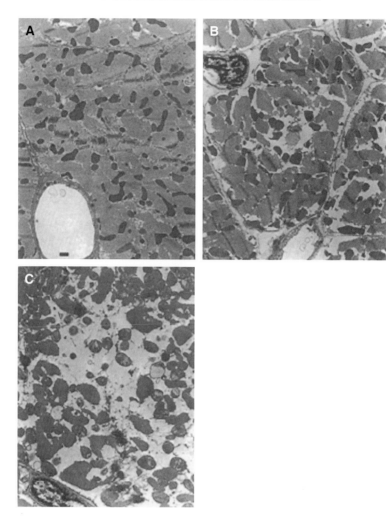

Fig. 2. Electron micrographs from (*A*) a normal dog, (*B*) a dog with MR and preserved LV function, and (*C*) a dog with MR and severe LV dysfunction. Note the progressive loss of contractile elements. (*From* Urabe Y, Mann DL, Kent RL, et al. Cellular and ventricular dysfunction in experimental canine mitral regurgitation. Circ Res 1992;70(1):141; with permission.)

coupling has also been noted [11]. This loss of contractile elements results in reduced mechanical function of the sarcomeres, with reduced sarcomere shortening and velocity of shortening at any given work load.

Insufficient hypertrophy of the myocytes has also been proposed as a mechanism of eventual LV failure. Unlike patients who have pressure overload in whom mass greatly exceeds volume, in patients who have MR, the ratio of mass to volume is less than 1. Thus, the increase in LV wall stress that accompanies the increase in LV volume is not associated with an appropriate hypertrophic response to normalize wall stress.

The increased systolic wall stress further taxes the left ventricle's contractile elements [5].

β-Adrenergic stimulation is a compensatory mechanism in all forms of heart failure that results in increased LV contractility and stroke volume. Over time, however, excessive β-adrenergic stimulation contributes to the decline in LV function. There is evidence of increased sympathetic nervous system activity in chronic MR [12,13]. Tstutsui and colleagues [14] demonstrated in an experimental dog model of MR that 3 months of treatment with the β-adrenergic blocker atenolol resulted in normalization of LV function. Normalization of structure was also noted at the cellular level. These findings suggest that adrenergic stimulation can be pathologic and contributes to the development of LV dysfunction and that β-blockade may be beneficial clinically, although this concept is yet to be tested in clinical trials [15]. Nemoto and colleagues [16] also demonstrated that normalization of LV function occurred after the administration of atenolol, whereas this effect was not noted when the angiotensin-receptor blocker lisinopril was used alone.

Despite the development of LV dysfunction and loss of contractile elements, improvement in LV function is often noted after surgical correction, suggesting that the maladaptive changes are not irreversible if treated early enough [17–19] and if the subvalvular apparatus is spared [18].

Unlike primary MR, which develops as a result of abnormalities in the mitral valve leaflets, secondary (or functional) MR develops as a consequence of LV dysfunction. The added volume overload imposed by MR contributes to further LV dilatation, progressive systolic dysfunction, and the development of more advanced heart failure. In keeping with this concept, a number of cohort studies have shown that patients who have LV dysfunction and MR have a worse outcome, in terms of survival and hospital admissions for heart failure, than patients who do not have MR (Fig. 3) [20–25]. Functional MR results because altered geometry of the LV [26,27] causes alteration of the mitral valve apparatus, leading to tethering of the mitral leaflets and abnormal leaflet coaptation [3,4,28,29]. "Ischemic" MR is most often the result of progressive postinfarct LV

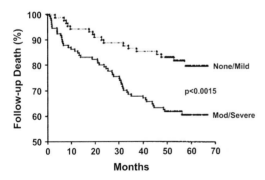

Fig. 3. Time to death according to the severity of MR in patients who had chronic systolic heart failure. Note the significant increase in mortality in those who had moderate (Mod) or severe MR. (*From* Robbins JD, Maniar PB, Cotts W, et al. Prevalence and severity of mitral regurgitation in chronic systolic heart failure. Am J Cardiol 2003;91:361; with permission.)

remodeling, rather than of ischemia. Because the mitral valve is attached to the left ventricle by way of the chords and papillary muscles, any alteration in loading conditions resulting in a change in the size or shape of the left ventricle can affect valve closure and thus the degree of regurgitation. Thus, medical therapies that improve LV remodeling tend to reduce the severity of functional MR [30–32], whereas factors that adversely affect loading conditions, such as hypertension, exacerbate MR and its impact on the left ventricle. Lancellotti and colleagues [33] found that patients who had coronary artery disease and LV dysfunction with significant MR at rest or who demonstrated an increase in MR severity with exercise were at greater risk of future morbidity and mortality (Fig. 4). Thus, in functional MR, evaluation of MR at rest alone may be insufficient to fully assess this disorder.

Unlike primary MR in which changes in LV function occur in a symmetric fashion, ischemic MR is much more complex due to associated postinfarct remodeling and other complications associated with coronary artery disease. Thus, focusing on the MR alone may be insufficient to adequately treat this problem. Guy and colleagues [34] showed that a prophylactic ventricular restraint device in sheep that had myocardial infarction reduced infarct expansion, attenuated adverse remodeling, and decreased ischemic MR, whereas mitral valve repair alone did not affect remodeling. Thus, ischemic MR is a consequence not a cause of postinfarction remodeling. This study implies that infarct expansion is an important therapeutic target.

Although extensive treatment guidelines exist [35] to assist in managing patients who have MR, the complexities of the hemodynamics and compensatory mechanisms in chronic MR and the absence of prospective randomized clinical trials result in continued difficulty for clinicians to appropriately time surgical correction in these patients.

Aortic regurgitation

AR can result from a number of pathologic disorders of the aortic valve or the aortic root [36]. Common etiologies affecting the valve include congenital disorders (especially bicuspid valves), calcific degenerative valves, systemic hypertension, rheumatic heart disease, infective endocarditis, and myxomatous degeneration. Bicuspid aortic valves are often associated with severe dilatation of the

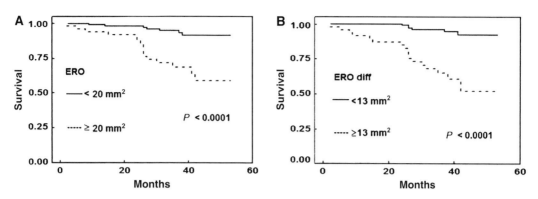

Fig. 4. Survival curves at rest (*A*) and during exercise (*B*). ERO, effective regurgitant orifice; diff, difference. (*From* Lancellotti P, Gerard PL, Pierard LA. Long term outcome of patients with heart failure and dynamic functional mitral regurgitation. Eur Heart J 2005;26:1530; with permission.)

aortic root and ascending aorta [37–39]. Other common disorders of the aortic root leading to AR include idiopathic dilatation, Marfan syndrome, or aortic dissection. Less common causes of AR include traumatic injuries to the aortic valve, ankylosing spondylitis, syphilitic aortitis, rheumatoid arthritis, discrete subaortic stenosis, and ventricular septal defects with prolapse of an aortic cusp [40]. Understanding the etiology of the regurgitation has important treatment implications, particularly if aortic root involvement is present.

Mechanisms of compensation for volume overload

Although MR and AR both result in volume overload of the left ventricle, the two lesions result in very different loading conditions. In AR, the sum of the regurgitant volume and the forward stroke volume is ejected into the aorta during systole, and the resultant increase in total ejected stroke volume creates systolic hypertension. In addition, the increased diastolic volume causes an increase in LV wall stress that must be overcome before systolic shortening can occur. The combination of systolic hypertension and increased LV wall stress results in a significant increase in LV afterload. Thus, in AR, there is volume overload and pressure overload. The volume overload results in compensatory eccentric hypertrophy, whereas the pressure overload results in superimposed concentric hypertrophy. The compensatory hypertrophy tends to normalize the mass-to-volume ratio, at least in the compensated stages of the disease. Through chamber dilatation, the left ventricle accommodates the increased end-diastolic volume without an increase in end-diastolic pressure. The addition

of new sarcomeres and the development of eccentric hypertrophy result in normalization of preload at the sarcomere level [41]. Thus, the left ventricle is able to maintain its preload reserve and normal performance of each contractile unit along the enlarged circumference. The end result is the ability to chronically maintain the augmented total stroke volume. As the disease progresses, increased systolic wall stress and afterload is a stimulus for further concentric hypertrophy that allows the left ventricle to maintain normal ejection performance despite increases in chamber volume and afterload.

These compensatory mechanisms often allow patients to remain asymptomatic for decades despite severe regurgitation. If preload reserve or compensatory hypertrophy is inadequate, however, further increases in afterload result in afterload mismatch, with a reduction in systolic performance and subsequent reduction in ejection fraction [41]. The resultant increase in LV filling pressures can result in symptoms of dyspnea and fatigue. Exertional angina can also develop as a result of diminished coronary flow reserve in the hypertrophied myocardium [42]. The transition from compensation to decompensation may occur slowly such that some patients may not present with symptoms until severe LV dysfunction develops. Depressed LV ejection fraction is initially a reversible process due to the afterload mismatch. If left untreated, however, progressive LV enlargement and remodeling develop and contractile dysfunction may occur. At this phase, patients are at risk for irreversible LV dysfunction even if surgical correction is undertaken (Fig. 5) [43].

The progression to irreversible LV dysfunction also occurs with changes in the myocardial

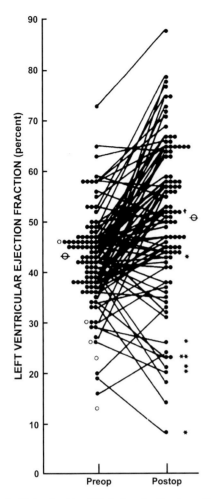

Fig. 5. Plots of resting LV ejection fraction by radionuclide angiography before (preop) and after (postop) aortic valve replacement. Open circles indicate patients who died before their 6-month evaluation, asterisks indicates patients who died from heart failure after the 6-month study, and the cross indicates one patient who died suddenly after 6 months. (*From* Bonow RO. Radionuclide angiography in the management of aortic regurgitation. Circulation 1991;84(Suppl I):I297; with permission.)

interstitium, with an increase in collagen and noncollagen connective tissue. Borer and colleagues [44] demonstrated that cardiac fibroblasts produce abnormal amounts of noncollagen extracellular matrix proteins, especially fibronectin, in animal models of AR and in patients who have this condition [45]. As with MR, the net accumulation of matrix proteins appears to result not from an increase in production but from a reduced rate of degradation of these proteins. Whether this

contributes to the demise of the left ventricle remains to be determined.

Compensatory mechanisms may also occur at the level of the arterial system. Devlin and colleagues [46] evaluated arterial elastance in patients who had AR plus compensated or decompensated LV function. They concluded that ideally, LV contractility and LV-arterial coupling are maintained in a range to maintain optimum mechanical efficiency. When LV contractile dysfunction develops, the arterial system may respond by decreasing elastance to maximize LV work. In some patients who have AR, arterial elastance may increase instead, resulting in an additional load on the left ventricle and subsequent reduction in LV pump efficiency.

The adaptive mechanisms for the left ventricle in chronic AR often result in the patient remaining asymptomatic for several years. Because symptoms may develop late after the development of LV dysfunction, close follow-up, including serial echocardiograms, is warranted to surgically correct the regurgitation before irreparable damage ensues [35].

Summary

AR and MR are two disorders in which the only similarities are the resultant volume overload of the left ventricle and the potential for irreversible LV systolic dysfunction before the onset of severe symptoms. In the compensated phase of MR, there is increased preload and normal afterload. The left ventricle compensates by undergoing enlargement and very little hypertrophy. These hemodynamic alterations associated with increased preload result in preserved ejection fraction even when contractile dysfunction develops. In contrast, AR results in increased preload and increased afterload, resulting in eccentric and concentric hypertrophy. Patients may remain asymptomatic for years until afterload mismatch results in LV dysfunction that is initially reversible. If left untreated, LV dysfunction in MR and AR may become irreversible [47]. Understanding the adaptive changes that the left ventricle undergoes in these volume-overload conditions has resulted in treatment guidelines to assist clinicians in timing of surgical correction.

Acknowledgments

The authors thank Juliet Robinson and Angelene Delk for their administrative and secretarial assistance.

References

[1] Otto CM. Evaluation and management of chronic mitral regurgitation. N Engl J Med 2001;345:740–6.

[2] Carabello BA. Mitral valve regurgitation. Curr Probl Cardiol 1998;23(4):200–41.

[3] Levine RA. Dynamic mitral regurgitation—more than meets the eye. N Engl J Med 2004;351: 1681–4.

[4] Levine RA, Schwammenthal E. Ischemic mitral regurgitation on the threshold of a solution: from paradoxes to unifying concepts. Circulation 2005; 112:745–58.

[5] Carabello BA. Progress in mitral and aortic regurgitation. Prog Cardiovasc Dis 2001;43:457–75.

[6] Imamura T, McDermott PJ, Kent RL, et al. Acute changes in myosin heavy chain synthesis rate in pressure vs volume overload. Circ Res 1994;75: 418–25.

[7] Matsuo T, Carabello BA, Nagatomo Y, et al. Mechanisms of cardiac hypertrophy in canine volume overload. Am J Physiol 1998;275:H65–74.

[8] Mulieri LA, Leavitt BJ, Ittleman FP, et al. Forskolin reverses the force-frequency defect in left ventricular subepicardium and (EPI) but not in papillary myocardium in mitral regurgitation heart failure. Circulation 1993;88(Suppl 1):406 [abstract].

[9] Spinale FG, Ishihara K, Zile M, et al. Structural basis for changes in left ventricular function and geometry because of chronic mitral regurgitation and after correction of volume overload. J Thorac Cardiovasc Surg 1993;106:1147–57.

[10] Urabe Y, Mann DL, Kent RL, et al. Cellular and ventricular dysfunction in experimental canine mitral regurgitation. Circ Res 1992;70(1):131–47.

[11] Mulieri LA, Leavitt BJ, Martin BJ, et al. Myocardial force frequency defect in mitral regurgitation heart failure is reversed by forskolin. Circulation 1998; 88:2700–4.

[12] Mehta RH, Supiano MA, Grossman PA, et al. Changes in systemic sympathetic nervous system activity after mitral valve surgery and their relationship to changes in left ventricular size and systolic performance in patients with mitral regurgitation. Am Heart J 2004;147:729–35.

[13] Mehta RH, Supiano MA, Oral H, et al. Compared with control subjects, the systemic sympathetic nervous system is activated in patients with mitral regurgitation. Am Heart J 2003;145:1078–85.

[14] Tsutsui H, Spinale FG, Nagatsu M, et al. Effects of chronic B-adrenergic blockade on the left ventricular and cardiocyte abnormalities of chronic canine mitral regurgitation. J Clin Invest 1994;93(6):2639–48.

[15] Starling MR. Is prophylactic beta-adrenergic blockade appropriate in mitral regurgitation: impact of cellular pathophysiology. Adv Cardiol 2004;41: 25–35.

[16] Nemoto S, Hamawaki M, De Freitas G, et al. Differential effects of angiotensin converting enzyme inhibitor lisinopril versus the β-adrenergic receptor blocker atenolol on hemodynamics and left ventricular contractile function in experimental mitral regurgitation. J Am Coll Cardiol 2002;40(1):149–54.

[17] Nakano K, Swindle MM, Spinale F, et al. Depressed contractile function due to canine mitral regurgitation improves after correction of volume overload. J Clin Invest 1991;87:2077–86.

[18] Ishihara K, Zile MR, Kanazawa S, et al. Left ventricular mechanics and myocyte function after correction of experimental chronic mitral regurgitation by combined mitral valve replacement and preservation of the native mitral valve apparatus. Circulation 1992;86(Suppl II):16–25.

[19] Starling MR. Effects of valve surgery on left ventricular contractile function in patients with long term mitral regurgitation. Circulation 1995;92:811–8.

[20] Robbins JD, Maniar PB, Cotts W, et al. Prevalence and severity of mitral regurgitation in chronic systolic heart failure. Am J Cardiol 2003;91:360–2.

[21] Trichon BH, Felker GM, Shaw LK, et al. Relation of frequency and severity of mitral regurgitation to survival among patients with left ventricular systolic dysfunction and heart failure. Am J Cardiol 2003;91: 538–43.

[22] Koelling TM, Aaronson KD, Cody RJ, et al. Prognostic significance of mitral regurgitation and tricuspid regurgitation in patients with left ventricular systolic dysfunction. Am Heart J 2002;144: 524–9.

[23] Grayburn PA, Appleton CP, DeMaria AN, et al. Echocardiographic predictors of morbidity and mortality in patients with advanced heart failure: the Beta-blocker Evaluation of Survival Trial (BEST). J Am Coll Cardiol 2005;45:1064–71.

[24] Grigioni F, Enriquez-Sarano M, Zehr KR, et al. Ischemic mitral regurgitation: long term outcome and prognostic implications with quantitative Doppler assessment. Circulation 2001;103:1759–64.

[25] Bursi F, Enriquez-Sarano M, Vuyisile TN, et al. Heart failure and death after myocardial infarction in the community: the emerging role of mitral regurgitation. Circulation 2005;111:295–301.

[26] Kono T, Sabbah HN, Rosman H, et al. Left ventricular shape is the primary determinant of functional mitral regurgitation in heart failure. J Am Coll Cardiol 1992;20:1594–8.

[27] Sabbah HN, Rosman H, Kono T, et al. On the mechanism of functional mitral regurgitation. Am J Cardiol 1993;72:1074–6.

[28] Karagiannis SE, Karatasakis GT, Koutsogiannis N, et al. Increased distance between mitral valve coaptation point and mitral annular plane: significance and correlations in patients with heart failure. Heart 2003;89:1174–8.

[29] Nielsen SL, Nygaard H, Mandrup L, et al. Mechanism of incomplete mitral leaflet coaptation—interaction of chordal restraint and changes in mitral leaflet coaptation geometry. Insight from in vitro

validation of the premise of force equilibrium. J Biomech Eng 2002;124:596–608.

[30] Capomolla S, Febo O, Gnemmi M, et al. β-Blockade therapy in chronic heart failure: diastolic function and mitral regurgitation improvement by carvedilol. Am Heart J 2000;139:596–608.

[31] St. John Sutton MG, Plappert T, Abraham WT, et al. Effect of cardiac resynchronization therapy on left ventricular size and function in chronic heart failure. Circulation 2003;107:1985–90.

[32] Breithardt OA, Sinha AM, Schwammenthal E, et al. Acute effects if cardiac resynchronization therapy on functional mitral regurgitation in advanced heart failure. J Am Coll Cardiol 2003;41:765–70.

[33] Lancellotti P, Gerard PL, Pierard LA. Long term outcome of patients with heart failure and dynamic functional mitral regurgitation. Eur Heart J 2005; 26:1528–32.

[34] Guy TS, Moaini SL, Gorman JH, et al. Prevention of ischemic mitral regurgitation does not influence the outcome of remodeling after posterolateral myocardial infarction. J Am Coll Cardiol 2004;43: 377–83.

[35] Bonow RO, Carabello BA, Kanu C, et al. ACC/AHA 2006 guidelines for the management of patients with valvular heart disease: a report of the American College of Cardiology/American Heart Association Task Force on Practice Guidelines (Writing Committee to Revise the 1998 Guidelines for the Management of Patients with Valvular Heart Disease) developed in collaboration with the Society of Cardiovascular Anesthesiologists; endorsed by the Society for Cardiovascular Angiography and Interventions and the Society of Thoracic Surgeons. Circulation 2006;114(5):e84–231.

[36] Roberts WC, Ko JM, Moore TR, et al. Causes of pure aortic regurgitation in patients having isolated aortic valve replacement at a single US tertiary hospital (1993 to 2005). Circulation 2006;114:422–9.

[37] Nistri S, Sorbo MD, Marin M, et al. Aortic root dilatation in young men with normally functioning bicuspid aortic valves. Heart 1999;82:19–22.

[38] Keane MG, Wiegers SE, Plappert T, et al. Bicuspid aortic valves are associated with aortic dilatation out of proportion to coexistent valvular lesions. Circulation 2000;102:III35–9.

[39] Braverman AC, Guven H, Beardslee MA, et al. The bicuspid aortic valve. Curr Probl Cardiol 2005;30: 470–522.

[40] Bonow RO. Aortic regurgitation. In: Zipes D, editor. Braunwald's heart disease: a textbook of cardiovascular medicine. Valvular heart disease, vol. 2. 7th edition. Philadelphia: WB Saunders; 2005. p. 1553–632.

[41] Bonow RO. Chronic aortic regurgitation. Cardiol Clin 1998;16(3):449–61.

[42] Nitenberg A, Foult JM, Antony I, et al. Coronary flow and resistance reserve in patients with chronic aortic regurgitation, angina pectoris and normal coronary arteries. J Am Coll Cardiol 1988;11:478–86.

[43] Bonow RO. Radionuclide angiography in the management of aortic regurgitation. Circulation 1991; 84(Suppl I):I296–302.

[44] Borer JS, Truter S, Herrold EM, et al. Myocardial fibrosis in chronic aortic regurgitation: molecular and cellular responses to volume overload. Circulation 2002;105:1837–42.

[45] Gupta A, Carter JN, Truter SL, et al. Cellular response of human cardiac fibroblasts to mechanically stimulated aortic regurgitation. Am J Ther 2006;13: 8–11.

[46] Devlin WH, Petrusha J, Briesmiester BS, et al. Impact of vascular adaptation to chronic aortic regurgitation on left ventricular performance. Circulation 1999;99:1027–33.

[47] Borer JS, Bonow RO. Contemporary approach to aortic and mitral regurgitation. Circulation 2003; 108:2432–8.

ELSEVIER
SAUNDERS

Heart Failure Clin 2 (2006) 461–471

HEART
FAILURE
CLINICS

Optimal Timing of Surgery in Aortic Regurgitation

William J. Stewart, MD, FACC, FASE[a,b,*]

[a]The Cleveland Clinic Foundation, Cleveland, OH, USA
[b]Cleveland Clinic Levner College of Medicine, Cleveland, OH, USA

Criteria for choosing the optimum time for operation in patients who have aortic regurgitation (AR) have changed in recent years, including a number of notable new components [1,2]. In the 1970s and 1980s, selecting patients for valvular surgery entailed waiting as long as possible until symptoms became substantial [3], which usually meant New York Heart Association (NYHA) class III symptoms that were not controllable with medical management. At that time, the primary surgical option was aortic valve replacement for which the perioperative mortality was high and postoperative problems with "prosthetic valve diseases" were substantial. In stable patients, clinicians watched for measurements of left ventricular (LV) size and function as the primary clinical indicators for surgical timing.

In current medical practice, the process of selecting patients is different in a variety of ways. Improved diagnostic methods are available to understand changes in the structure of the aortic valve itself, often including the etiology and mechanism of the dysfunction. Acute cardiac imaging allows a better understanding of a patient's aortic valve and allows better prediction of the likely future progression of the disease based on natural history studies. Improved quantitation of the severity of the AR is feasible using Doppler echocardiography and other methods. The effects of AR on cardiac function and the potential complications that occur with medical or surgical management can be anticipated. Operative mortality has declined remarkably. For isolated, uncomplicated aortic valve operations at Cleveland Clinic, in-hospital mortality decreased from 2.4% during 1980 to 1989 to 1.7% during 1990 to 1999 and to 1.2% during 2000 to 2005. Surgical options have improved, including more nonprosthetic options such as valve repair. Available prosthetic valves are more durable than in the past. In patients needing isolated primary aortic valve surgery, minimally invasive techniques [4] can be used, avoiding some the discomfort, bleeding, and other temporary disabilities resulting from a full midsternal thoracotomy. Newly developed percutaneous [5–7] and robotic [8] methods have already been used in limited numbers of patients, and their future role is hopeful.

Accordingly, the threshold for valve surgery has been progressively reduced. It is now reasonable to do valve surgery for AR in some asymptomatic patients. The clinician must carefully consider each patient individually, including his or her current state of health and fitness, all noncardiology problems, and the available resources for medical treatment, surgery, and recovery. Decisions for surgery or medical management should be based on a comparison between the likely outcomes of immediate surgery and the natural history of the disease if surgery is delayed.

Mechanisms and etiologies of aortic regurgitation

The mechanisms of AR can be determined with good accuracy by echocardiography [9,10]. An excellent paradigm is to categorize AR by its association with aortic leaflet motion that is normal, excessive, or restricted (Fig. 1). The pattern of leaflet motion impacts on the surgical options and reflects the amount to which the disease

* Department of Cardiovascular Medicine, The Cleveland Clinic Foundation, 9500 Euclid Avenue, Desk F-15, Cleveland, OH 44195.
 E-mail address: stewarw@ccf.org

1551-7136/06/$ - see front matter © 2007 Elsevier Inc. All rights reserved.
doi:10.1016/j.hfc.2006.09.007

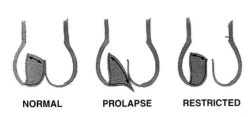

NORMAL   PROLAPSE   RESTRICTED

Fig. 1. Mechanistic understanding of AR based on leaflet motion. AR can result from normal leaflet motion (*left*) due to dilated aortic root or leaflet perforation, excessive leaflet motion (*center*) due to prolapse of a redundant or bileaflet valve, or restricted leaflet motion (*right*) due to fibrosis and calcification. (*From* Cosgrove DM, Rosenkranz ER, Hendren WG, et al. Valvuloplasty for aortic insufficiency. J Thorac Cardiovasc Surg 1991; 102:571–6; with permission. Copyright © 1991, American Association for Thoracic Surgery.)

process has affected the size and integrity of the leaflet tissue and its suspension. For example, in a patient whose ascending aorta is enlarging, the aortic valve is normal even though its suspension is abnormal. As the sinotubular junction is displaced outward and upward, the normal aortic leaflets no longer coapt in the middle, and central AR results.

The causes of AR include calcific degeneration, congenital disease, rheumatic disease, aortic aneurysms and dissection, infective endocarditis, aortitis, myxomatous disease, anorectic drugs, connective tissue diseases like lupus erythematosis, Marfan syndrome, trauma, and others. Each of these etiologies may cause a range of effects on the aortic valve and its supporting apparatus (Fig. 2). The most common disease process

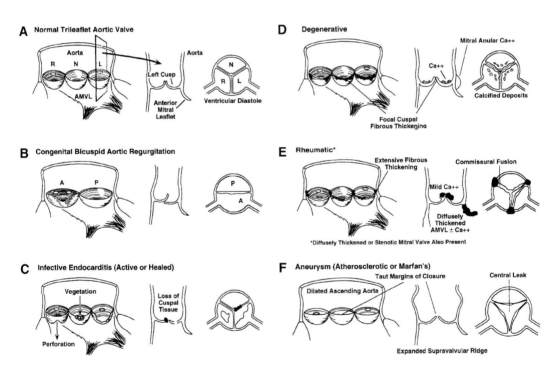

Fig. 2. Diagrams showing various etiologies of AR. Each of the six panels shows a long axis of the aortic root opened up to show all the leaflets (*left*), a schematic of the long axis of the sinus of Valsalva (*center*), and a schematic of the short axis of the aortic valve (*right*). (*A*) Normal trileaflet aortic valve. (*B*) Congenital bicuspid valve with a raphe between what would be the right and left coronary cusps in an anterior cusp that is larger than the posterior cusp, causing prolapse and AR. (*C*) Endocarditis causes AR through disruption of valve suspension or leaflet perforation. (*D*) Degenerative changes cause AR by restricting leaflet motion and coaptation. (*E*) Rheumatic valvulitis causes AR with postinflammatory leaflet fusion and fibrosis. (*F*) Aneurysms from atherosclerosis or cystic medial necrosis (Marfan type) cause AR by outward displacement of the leaflet suspension with central noncoaptation or by dissection, causing failure of leaflet support. A, anterior; AMVL, anterior mitral valve leaflet coronary cusp; Ca++, calcification; L, left; N, noncoronary cusp; P, posterior; R, right coronary cusp. (*Modified from* Waller BF. Evaluation of operatively excised cardiac valves. Contemporary Issues in Cardiovascular Pathology. Cardiovasc Clin 1998;18(2):220; with permission.)

causing aortic valve disease in the Western world is an atherosclerotic process that causes degenerative fibrosis, thickening, and calcification of the aortic leaflets, similar to the pathology that causes coronary and peripheral vascular atherosclerosis [11]. In most patients who have this disease and need valve surgery, the most common valve dysfunction is aortic stenosis, but some patients who have fibrocalcific disease present with AR.

Surgical options in aortic regurgitation

Surgery in a patient who has AR may entail a stented bovine pericardial bioprosthesis, a mechanical prosthesis, valve repair, an aortic homograft, a stentless porcine bioprosthesis, a stented porcine bioprosthesis, or the Ross procedure (a pulmonary autograft plus a pulmonary homograft). Each option has some advantages and disadvantages, especially with respect to its feasibility, availability, durability, and risks of failure [12]. In recent years, mechanical prosthetic valves have declined in popularity due to the travails of anticoagulation and the morbidity (during the entire life of the prosthesis) of bleeding and clotting events. Also contributing to this trend is the

improved durability of bovine bioprostheses, which usually last longer than 20 years—better than their porcine predecessors. In the future when percutaneous valve replacement is more feasible, it is likely to be more applicable to patients who have previous bioprostheses than those who have mechanical prostheses.

Valve repair is a good option primarily for two specialized morphologic groups. The first includes patients who have noncalcified prolapsing valves [13]. These valves are usually congenital bicuspid valves, having two leaflets in which the AR results from prolapse [14] because one of the leaflets (the larger conjoined one) has a longer leaflet edge than the other. The second type of AR amenable to repair is found in the patients previously mentioned, who have normal leaflets that are tethered outward by dilation of the ascending aorta, or annular dilation [10].

Quantitation of aortic regurgitation

As many as seven methods using Doppler echocardiography are used in tandem to derive a summary assessment of the severity of AR (Fig. 3, Table 1) [15]. MRI and angiography [16]

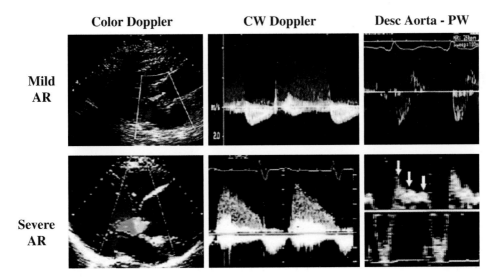

Fig. 3. Methods of quantitation of AR. Mild AR (*upper row*) is exemplified by a color Doppler jet with a diameter less than 10% of the diameter of the LV outflow tract diameter (*left*), a continuous wave (CW) Doppler showing diastolic density far less than the systolic density with a long pressure half-time (*center*), and only brief diastolic flow reversal in the descending aorta (*right*). Severe AR (*lower row*) is evidenced by a wide color jet with a diameter greater than 65% of the LV outflow tract diameter (*left*), a CW Doppler showing diastolic density equal to the density of the systolic signal with a short pressure half-time (*center*), and pandiastolic flow reversal (*arrows*) in the descending aorta (*right*). (*From* Zoghbi WA, Enriquez-Sarano M, Foster E, et al. Recommendations for evaluation of the severity of native valvular regurgitation with two-dimensional and Doppler echocardiography. J Am Soc Echocardiogr 2003;16:777–802; with permission. Copyright © 2003, American Society of Echocardiography.)

Table 1
Qualitative and quantitative parameters useful in grading aortic regurgitation severity

Parameters	Mild	Moderate/moderate to severe	Severe
Structural			
LA size	Normal[a]	Normal or dilated	Usually dilated[b]
Aortic leaflets	Normal or abnormal	Normal or abnormal	Abnormal/flail or wide coaptation defect
Doppler			
Jet width in LVOT—color flow	Small in central jets	Intermediate	Large in central jets; variable in eccentric jets
Jet density–CW	Incomplete or faint	Dense	Dense
Jet deceleration rate–CW (PHT)[c]	Slow >500	Medium 500–200	Steep <200
Diastolic flow reversal in descending aorta–PW	Brief, early diastolic reversal	Intermediate	Prominent holodiastolic reversal
Quantitative[d]			
VC width (cm)[e]	<0.3	0.3–0.60	>0.6
Jet width/LVOT width (%)[e]	<25	25–45/46–64	≥65
Jet CSA/LVOT CSA (%)[e]	<5	5–20/21–59	≥60
R Vol (mL/beat)	<30	30–44/45–59	≥60
RF (%)	<30	30–39/40–49	≥50
EROA (cm^2)	<0.10	0.10–0.19/0.20–0.29	≥0.30

Abbreviations: CSA, cross-sectional area; CW, continuous wave Doppler; EROA, effective regurgitant orifice area; LA, left atrium; LVOT, LV outflow tract; PHT, pressure half-time; PW, pulsed wave Doppler; R Vol, regurgitant volume; RF, regurgitant fraction; VC, vena contracta.

[a] Unless there are other reasons for LV dilation. Normal two-dimensional measurements: LV minor axis ≤2.8 cm/m^2, LV end-diastolic volume ≤82 ml/m^2.

[b] Exception would be acute AR, in which chambers have not had time to dilate.

[c] PHT, measured in milliseconds, is shortened with increasing LV diastolic pressure and vasodilator therapy and may be lengthened in chronic adaptation to severe AR.

[d] Quantitative parameters can subclassify the moderate regurgitation group into moderate and moderate-to-severe regurgitation as shown.

[e] At a Nyquist limit of 50–60 cm/s.

Data from Zoghbi WA, Enriquez-Sarano M, Foster E, et al. Recommendations for evaluation of the severity of native valvular regurgitation with two-dimensional and Doppler echocardiography. J Am Soc Echocardiogr 2003;16:777–802.

are used occasionally, especially in equivocal cases. The most widely used ultrasound method uses the width of color Doppler aliasing of the proximal AR jet [17] expressed as a percentage of the diameter of the LV outflow tract (LVOT), although this measure is problematic when the jet is eccentric in direction or nontubular in shape. Pulsed Doppler echocardiography can evaluate the degree of diastolic reversal in the descending aorta caused by the backflow of blood into the left ventricle. A continuous wave (CW) Doppler recording can evaluate the pressure half-time of the AR diastolic maximum velocity, reflecting the decay in the pressure difference between aortic and LV pressures. The density of the same CW Doppler recording compared with the antegrade signal density is another useful method, although it is subjective. Other types of "spatial mapping" options assess the area of color Doppler aliasing of the AR jet in a short axis view of the LVOT, or the amount to which the diastolic aliasing extends toward the LV apex. Flow can be measured quantitatively based on the aliasing radius of the color Doppler flow convergence (Fig. 4) on the aortic side of the regurgitant orifice using a formula based on hemispheric geometry of this velocity field and the continuity of diastolic flow through the orifice (Fig. 5). Combined with the maximum velocity measured by CW Doppler, the regurgitant orifice area can be calculated

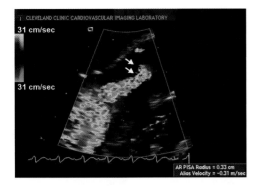

Fig. 4. Color Doppler stop-frame image of the largest obtainable jet in a patient who had mild AR, recorded at a Nyquist level of 31 cm/s. The aliasing radius of the flow convergence on the aortic side of the jet is measured from the upper arrow (at the blue-yellow interface) to the lower arrow (at the jet orifice, the smallest diameter of the jet). Using a maximum velocity of 400 cm/s (recorded by CW Doppler, not shown), the calculated maximum instantaneous orifice area would be 0.05 cm², which is mild AR. Note that the size of the jet would have been much smaller if the color Doppler were recorded at a Nyquist level of 50 to 60 cm/s, the setting usually used for spatial mapping.

[18,19]. The area under the CW recording of the AR signal, representing the stroke distance, can be added to the formula to calculate regurgitant volume. The vena contracta method measures the minor diameter of color aliasing at the orifice itself (more proximal than the LVOT jet width mentioned earlier). The final way to measure AR is to compare quantitative estimates of antegrade flow through the LVOT and through the mitral annulus using the product of cross-sectional area and the integral of the pulsed Doppler velocity.

Natural history of acute and chronic aortic regurgitation

The natural history of AR and its likely effects on intracardiac pressure and LV size and function are cartooned in Fig. 6. The optimum management of a patient depends on understanding how far the person has gone along this course. Patients vary in the rapidity with which they progress along the natural history, in part due to the etiology, mechanism, and severity of their AR. The rapidity of progression also depends on how the patient's myocardium responds to the progression of the disease.

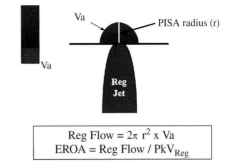

$$Reg\ Flow = 2\pi\ r^2\ x\ Va$$
$$EROA = Reg\ Flow\ /\ PkV_{Reg}$$

Fig. 5. Artistic diagram of the flow convergence method of quantitation of AR, based on the proximal isovelocity surface area (PISA) method. EROA, effective regurgitant orifice area; PkV$_{Reg}$, peak velocity of the regurgitant flow measured with CW Doppler; Reg, regurgitant; Va, aliasing velocity. (*Adapted from* Zoghbi WA, Enriquez-Sarano M, Foster E, et al. Recommendations for evaluation of the severity of native valvular regurgitation with two-dimensional and Doppler echocardiography. J Am Soc Echocardiogr 2003;16:777–802; with permission. Copyright © 2003, American Society of Echocardiography.)

If the onset of severe AR is rapid (see Fig. 6B) and the patient becomes extremely ill with acute pulmonary edema, then detection of AR may be difficult because many of the bedside findings of severe AR may be absent. There is a sudden and severe rise in LV diastolic pressure but relatively little change in aortic pressure or pulse contour. Forward stroke volume is reduced, so heart rate rises to preserve cardiac output. The left ventricle becomes hyperdynamic but cannot dilate acutely very much. Furthermore, the diastolic murmur of acute AR may be hard to hear because LV diastolic pressure is not much lower than aortic diastolic pressure.

When AR progresses more slowly (see Fig. 6C), LV diastolic volume increases substantially to accommodate the increased diastolic filling (volume overload). Because of systolic hypertension and compensatory increases in systemic resistance, LV pressure overload also occurs. To relieve the elevated wall stress, LV mass increases, causing eccentric and concentric LV hypertrophy with LV cavity dilation. The gradual LV adaptation maintains good diastolic compliance, keeping LV filling pressures normal or minimally elevated. The large total LV stroke volume allows forward stroke volume to be normal despite a large regurgitant volume. The result is an asymptomatic patient who has a compensated though severely dilated LV and a wide pulse pressure. These hemodynamics generate the "named

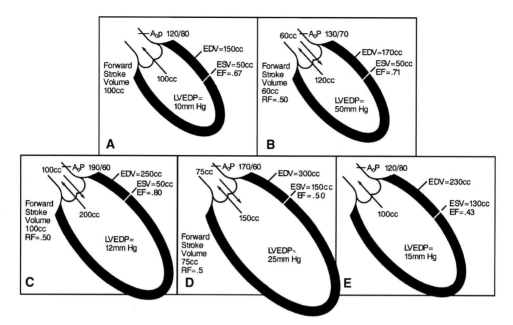

Fig. 6. Intracardiac pressure and volume hemodynamics of the clinical stages of AR. (*A*) Normal conditions. (*B*) Severe acute AR. Although total stroke volume (SV) is increased, forward SV is reduced. LV end-diastolic pressure (LVEDP) rises dramatically. (*C*) Chronic, compensated AR. Eccentric hypertrophy produces increased end-diastolic volume (EDV), which permits an increase in total and forward SV. The volume overload is accommodated, and LVEDP is normalized. Ventricular emptying and end-systolic volume (ESV) remain normal. (*D*) Chronic, decompensated AR. Impaired LV emptying produces an increase in ESV and a decrease in ejection fraction (EF), total SV, and forward SV. There is further cardiac dilation and recurrence of moderately elevated LVEDP. (*E*) Immediately after aortic valve replacement, preload estimated by EDV decreases, as does LVEDP. ESV is also decreased but to a lesser extent, resulting in an initial decrease in EF. Despite these changes, elimination of AR leads to an increase in forward SV. A_oP, aortic pressure; RF, regurgitant fraction. (*Modified from* Carabello BA. Aortic regurgitation: hemodynamic determinants of prognosis. In: Cohn LH, DiSesa VJ, editors. Aortic regurgitation: medical and surgical management. New York: Marcel Dekker; 1986; with permission.)

bedside findings," such as the Duroziez's sign (Table 2). The physiology of chronic AR differs markedly from mitral regurgitation, which usually has normal LV wall thickness, normal pulse pressure, and a pure LV volume overload without pressure overload.

After many years of significant AR (but sometimes much sooner), the uncorrected pathology may cause progressive LV failure and myocardial dysfunction (see Fig. 6D). Contractile dysfunction, depressed ejection fraction, and decreased diastolic compliance generate increased LV filling pressures. This chronic decompensated phase is reversible in its early phase but becomes irreversible as myocardial dysfunction progresses. Finally, if a patient undergoes aortic valve replacement before the onset of severe myocardial dysfunction, then adverse LV dynamics

revert toward normal or completely normalize (see Fig. 6E).

Predictors of myocardial dysfunction and adverse outcome in aortic regurgitation

From natural history studies of isolated severe AR [20,21], symptomatic patients who have severe AR and do not have corrective surgery suffer a mortality rate greater than 10% per year. In contrast, patients who have severe AR and are asymptomatic often do well over fairly long intervals, with an observed rate of sudden death of less than 0.2% per year. Therefore, it is not imperative to operate on a patient solely on the basis of severe AR if the person does not have symptoms, LV enlargement or dysfunction, dilation of the ascending aorta, rapid progression (including an

Table 2
Bedside findings of chronic severe aortic regurgitation

Sign	Finding
Duroziez's sign	Diastolic bruit over femoral artery when artery is partially compressed
Quincke's pulse	Systolic plethora and diastolic blanching in nail bed when nail is compressed
de Musset's sign	Bobbing of head
Corrigan's pulse	Rapid forceful carotid upstroke followed by rapid decline
Hill's sign	Augmentation of systolic pressure in leg by >30 mm Hg compared with arm

Data from Stewart WJ, Carabello BA. Aortic valve disease. In: Topol EJ, editor. Textbook of cardiovascular medicine. 2nd edition. Philadelphia: Lippincott, Williams and Wilkins; 2002.

unstable etiology like active endocarditis or acute aortic dissection), or other complications of the disease. In asymptomatic patients who have normal LV function, medical management should include careful surveillance for symptoms or significant LV abnormalities. The rate of progression to depressed LV ejection fraction (without symptoms) is less than 3.5% per year, and the rate of progression to symptoms (usually heart failure) without LV dysfunction is less than 6% per year. After a patient has developed systolic dysfunction, however, the rate of progression to cardiac symptoms is greater than 25% per year [2,20].

Numerous factors are predictive of reduced postoperative survival and poor recovery of LV function after surgery for AR. These factors include the severity of preoperative symptoms, reduced exercise tolerance, depression of myocardial function, and increase in ventricular chamber size. In asymptomatic patients, end-systolic cavity enlargement is a useful harbinger of underlying myocardial dysfunction. In contrast, depression of ejection fraction is sometimes a late and therefore unreliable finding because the chronic volume overload and high stroke volume artificially elevates the observed ejection fraction, hiding the appearance of decreased myocardial function until later in the course of the disease. Thus, end-systolic diameter or volume indices are more

preload-independent indices than ejection fraction and, therefore, more helpful in timing surgery [22].

Published guidelines on timing of surgery in aortic regurgitation

Recommendations for operative thresholds in patients who have AR have recently been updated (Fig. 7). Note that the decisions pivot on symptoms, exercise testing, LV ejection fraction, LV systolic dimensions, changes in LV dimensions, and serial evaluations. Any symptoms of congestive heart failure represent a class I indication for surgery (Box 1). Of note, there is recognition in the decision tree that some patients' symptoms are equivocal as to whether the symptoms result from the AR. Any depression of resting ejection fraction below the lower limit of normal (usually 55%) for the laboratory is also a class I indication for surgery. In addition, a systolic LV diameter greater than 55 mm in an average-sized male patient is a class I indication for surgery because studies suggest that postoperative survival is already significantly decreased [23]. A systolic LV diameter greater than 50 mm should be strongly considered for surgery unless there is a reassuring hemodynamic response to exercise. The generalization to women of the unadjusted LV diameter surgical criteria established in men, however, results in irrelevant criteria almost never reached by women [24]. This problem is not entirely avoided by correction of LV chamber dimensions by body surface area [22]. Exercise imaging is helpful to provide information on the "reserve strength" of the LV unmasked by exercise. Stress testing also allows direct observation of exercise tolerance and of severity and threshold for symptoms [21]. If surgery is performed within 1.5 years or so after reaching these LV sizes or ejection fraction thresholds, then myocardial function is still likely return to normal after postoperative remodeling [25], whereas prolonged LV abnormalities are more likely permanent.

Individual differences among patients in loading conditions and in the hemodynamic response to AR confound standard clinical indices of contractile dysfunction, such as ejection fraction. Serial re-evaluation at more frequent intervals is warranted when borderline symptoms, LV size, or exercise response is suspected. Diameters measured under varying loading conditions or at different laboratories using different angles to the LV shape may also lead to variations in diameter, volume, and ejection fraction, conveying trends

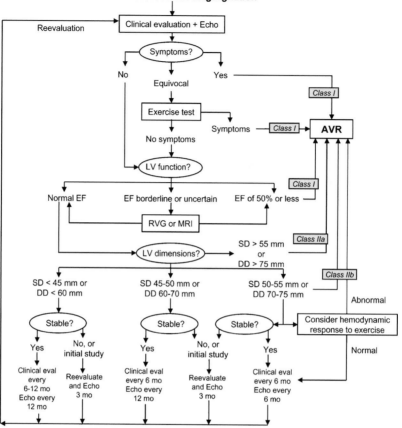

Fig. 7. Flow diagram representing guideline recommendations for management of AR, especially regarding the decision on timing of operative intervention. AVR, aortic valve replacement; Echo, echocardiography; EF, ejection fraction; DD, end-diastolic dimension; RVG, radionuclide ventriculography; SD, end-systolic diameter. (*From* Bonow RO, Carabello BA, Chatterjee K, et al. ACC/AHA 2006 guidelines for the management of patients with valvular heart disease, a report of the American College of Cardiology/American Heart Association Task Force on Practice Guidelines. J Am Coll Cardiol 2006;48:e1–148; with permission.)

that are not reflective of true clinical deterioration. Changes of less than 5 mm diameter or less than 5% ejection fraction are possibly within the error of the method.

For asymptomatic patients who are followed serially, the frequency of follow-up echocardiographic studies should be every 2 years when the end-systolic diameter is less than 40 mm and yearly when the end-systolic diameter is 40 to 50 mm.

Ascending aortic dilation

The health or disease of the ascending aorta represents another important parameter in following some patients who have AR. An ascending aortic aneurysm from atherosclerotic disease or cystic medial necrosis is a common etiology of AR. Size indicators for operation for the ascending aorta may develop before or after those for the valvular AR alone.

Approximately half of the patients who have a bicuspid valve develop an aortopathy resembling cystic medial necrosis, as seen in Marfan syndrome. The aorta of these patients tends to dilate progressively, independent of the persistence or surgical correction of the valvular process.

Dissection or spontaneous rupture of the aorta may be the first indicator of a thoracic aortic aneurysm. Patients who have large aneurysms and

Box 1. Summary of indications for surgery with severe aortic regurgitation

Symptoms >NYHA class II resulting from AR
- Exercise study to assess exercise capacity objectively

Abnormal LV size and function— (possibly adjusting for body surface area)
- Any contractile dysfunction (ejection fraction <55%) (percent fractional shortening <27%)
- Systolic LV internal diameter >50–55 mm
- Diastolic LV internal diameter >70–75 mm
- (Abnormal change in LV ejection fraction or LV end-systolic volume with exercise)

Enlarged ascending aorta (>5.0–5.5 cm diameter)

marfanoid women who become pregnant are particularly prone to aortic catastrophes. Emergent surgery in the setting of acute dissection has a 10 to 20 fold increase in mortality risk compared with elective operations. In patients whose aortic enlargement is discovered in an asymptomatic stage, the risk of subsequent aortic rupture or dissection increases with larger thoracic aorta diameter [26].

Patients who have ascending aortic dilation more than 5.5 cm should be considered for elective ascending aortic replacement. The threshold for surgery should be lower in the presence of significant AR and significant effacement of the shape of the sinotubular junction. The threshold should also be adjusted for body size, with women and smaller patients having elective surgery at a smaller size than larger men. One postulated threshold is to operate when the ratio of the patient's maximum aortic cross-sectional area in short axis (in centimeters squared) divided by the patient's height (in meters) is greater than 10 [27,28]. As an example, an aorta measuring 5.5 cm in diameter (cross-sectional area, 23.7 cm^2) in a 6-foot (1.84-m) tall patient represents a ratio of 12.9. In contrast, a ratio of 10 in a person 5 feet (1.54 m) tall would occur at a diameter of 4.5 cm (cross-sectional area, 15.9 cm^2). Height seems to be better as a criterion to gauge excessive

aortic size because it depends less on eating habits and the degree of obesity.

Standard surgical treatment for ascending aortic dilation is usually replacement with a hemashield graft. In many patients, the aortic valve is replaced with a prosthetic valve—biologic or mechanical. Some patients can have aortic valve resuspension with a supracoronary graft or a David procedure [29], which includes the lower anastamosis of the conduit right down at the aortic annulus, with reimplantation of the coronary arteries as buttons into the graft.

In a patient who has indications for surgery on the basis of an abnormal aortic valve and has an aortopathy, it seems reasonable to do preemptive aortic root replacement at a threshold slightly lower that that mentioned previously (eg, above an ascending aortic diameter of 4.5 cm). For the same reasons, after isolated surgery for a bicuspid aortic valve, patients should have serial CT or MRI evaluation every 2 to 5 years if there is any evidence of aortopathy.

Afterload reduction for medical treatment of aortic regurgitation

The optimum medical management strategy for AR has been reconsidered lately. A decade ago, several articles showed seemingly clear-cut improvement in outcome of groups of patients who had severe AR and who were treated with afterload-reducing medicines. For example, nifedipine-treated patients who had AR had better outcome than those treated with digoxin [30]. In contrast, a recent randomized study showed no improvement in AR patients treated with nifedipine or enalapril compared with placebo [31]. Thus, the long-held tenet that vasodilator therapy improves outcome in the presence of severe asymptomatic AR has been challenged by this recent prospective study. In contrast, medical management of asymptomatic patients who have ascending aortic dilation usually includes a negative inotropic agent like a β-blocker, which decreases the systolic shear rate in the aorta by reducing dp/dt (change in pressure per time).

Summary

Recommendations regarding the optimal timing for surgery in AR must be made individually for each patient based on benefits and risks of each approach. Aortic valve surgery should be recommended if the patient who has severe AR has any symptoms, if echocardiography demonstrates LV dysfunction (ejection fraction <55%), or an end-systolic diameter approaches 50 to 55 mm. The exercise response and other complicating factors should also be considered. The surgical options must be considered based on how the mechanism and the etiology of the AR (based on current imaging techniques) are likely to affect the natural history of the disease.

References

[1] Bonow RO, Carabello BA, Chatterjee K, et al. ACC/AHA 2006 guidelines for the management of patients with valvular heart disease, a report of the American College of Cardiology/American Heart Association Task Force on Practice Guidelines. J Am Coll Cardiol 2006;48:e1–148.

[2] Bonow RO, Carabello B, de Leon AC Jr, et al. Guidelines for the management of patients with valvular heart disease: executive summary. A report of the American College of Cardiology/American Heart Association Task Force on Practice Guidelines. Circulation 1998;98(18):1949–84.

[3] Assey ME, Usher BW, Carabello BA, et al. The patient with valvular heart disease. In: Pepine CJ, Hill JA, Lambert CR, editors. Diagnostic and therapeutic cardiac catheterization. 2nd edition. Baltimore: Williams & Wilkins; 1989. p. 471–507.

[4] Cosgrove DM, Sabik JF. Minimally invasive approach for aortic valve operations. Ann Thorac Surg 1996;62:596–7.

[5] Cribier A, Eltchaninoff H, Tron C, et al. Early experience with percutaneous transcatheter implantation of heart valve prosthesis for the treatment of end-stage inoperable patients with calcific aortic stenosis. J Am Coll Cardiol 2004;43(4):698–703.

[6] Webb JG, Chandavimol M, Thompson CR, et al. Percutaneous aortic valve implantation retrograde from the femoral artery. Circulation 2006;113(6): 842–50.

[7] Vassiliades TA Jr, Block PC, Cohn LH, et al. The clinical development of percutaneous heart valve technology: a position statement of the Society of Thoracic Surgeons (STS), the American Association for Thoracic Surgery (AATS), and the Society of Cardiovascular Angiography and Intervention (SCAI). J Am Coll Cardiol 2005;45(9): 1554–60.

[8] Folliguet TA, Vanhuyse F, Konstantinos Z, et al. Early experience with robotic aortic valve replacement. Eur J Cardiothorac Surg 2005;28(1):172–3.

[9] Cohen GI, Duffy CI, Klein AL, et al. Color Doppler and two-dimensional echocardiographic determination of the mechanism of aortic regurgitation with surgical correlation. J Am Soc Echocardiogr 1996; 9:508–15.

[10] Movsowitz HD, Levine RA, Hilgenberg AD, et al. Transesophageal description of the mechanisms of aortic regurgitation in acute type A aortic dissection—implications for aortic valve repair. J Am Coll Cardiol 2000;3:884–90.

[11] Otto CM, Kuusisto J, Reichenbach DD, et al. Characterization of the early lesion of "degenerative" valvular aortic stenosis: histological and immunohistochemical studies. Circulation 1994;90:844.

[12] Hammermeister K, Sethi GK, Henderson WG, et al. Outcomes 15 years after valve replacement with a mechanical versus a bioprosthetic valve: final report of the veterans affairs randomized trial. J Am Coll Cardiol 2000;36:1152–8.

[13] Cosgrove DM, Rosenkranz ER, Hendren WG, et al. Valvuloplasty for aortic insufficiency. J Thorac Cardiovasc Surg 1991;102:571–6.

[14] Stewart WJ, King ME, Weyman AE. Prevalence of aortic valve prolapse with bicuspid aortic valve and its relation to aortic regurgitation: a cross-sectional echocardiographic study. Am J Cardiol 1984;54:1277–82.

[15] Zoghbi WA, Enriquez-Sarano M, Foster E, et al. Recommendations for evaluation of the severity of native valvular regurgitation with two-dimensional and Doppler echocardiography. J Am Soc Echocardiogr 2003;16:777–802.

[16] Sellers RD, Levy MJ, Amplatz K. Left retrograde cardioangiography in acquired cardiac disease: technique, indications, and interpretations in 700 cases. Am J Cardiol 1964;14:437.

[17] Reynolds T, Abate J, Tenney A, et al. The JH/LVOH method in the quantification of aortic regurgitation: how the cardiac sonographer may avoid an important potential pitfall. J Am Soc Echocardiogr 1991;4:105–8.

[18] Tribouilloy CM, Enriquez-Sarano M, Fett SL, et al. Application of the proximal flow convergence method to calculate the effective regurgitant orifice area in aortic regurgitation. J Am Coll Cardiol 1998;32:1032–9.

[19] Shiota T, Jones M, Agler DA, et al. New echocardiographic windows for quantitative determination of aortic regurgitation volume using color Doppler flow convergence and vena contracta. Am J Cardiol 1999;83(7):1064–8.

[20] Bonow RO, Lakatos E, Maron BJ, et al. Serial long-term assessment of the natural history of asymptomatic patients with chronic aortic regurgitation and normal left ventricular systolic function. Circulation 1991;84:1625.

[21] Borer JS, Herrold EM, Hochreiter C, et al. Natural history of left ventricular performance at rest and during exercise after aortic valve replacement for aortic regurgitation. Circulation 1991;84(Suppl III): III133–9.

[22] Carabello BA, Usher BW, Hendrix GH, et al. Predictors of outcome for aortic valve replacement in patients with aortic regurgitation and left ventricular

dysfunction: a change in the measuring stick. J Am Coll Cardiol 1987;10:991.

[23] Henry WL, Bonow RO, Borer JS, et al. Observations on the optimum time for operative intervention for aortic regurgitation. I. Evaluation of the results of aortic valve replacement in symptomatic patients. Circulation 1980;61:471.

[24] Klodas E, Enriquez-Sarano M, Tajik AJ, et al. Surgery for aortic regurgitation in women. Contrasting indications and outcomes compared with men. Circulation 1996;94(10):2472–8.

[25] Bonow RO, Rosing DR, Maron BJ, et al. Reversal of left ventricular dysfunction after aortic valve replacement for chronic regurgitation: influence of duration of preoperative left ventricular dysfunction. Circulation 1984;70:570.

[26] Coady MA, Rizzo JA, Hammond GL, et al. What is the appropriate size criterion for resection of thoracic aortic aneurysms? J Thorac Cardiovasc Surg 1997;113(3):476–91.

[27] Svensson LG, Kim KH, Lytle BW, et al. Relationship of aortic cross-sectional area to height ratio and the risk of aortic dissection in patients with bicuspid aortic valves. J Thorac Cardiovasc Surg 2003;126(3):892–3.

[28] Svensson LG, Khitin L. Aortic cross-sectional area/height ratio timing of aortic surgery in asymptomatic patients with Marfan syndrome. J Thorac Cardiovasc Surg 2002;123(2):360–1.

[29] David TE, Feindel CM, Bos J. Repair of the aortic valve in patients with aortic insufficiency and aortic root aneurysm. J Thorac Cardiovasc Surg 1995;109:345–51.

[30] Scognamiglio R, Rahimtoola SH, Fasoli G, et al. Nifedipine in asymptomatic patients with severe aortic regurgitation and normal left ventricular function. N Engl J Med 1994;331:689.

[31] Evangelista A, Tornos P, Sambola A, et al. Long-term vasodilator therapy in patients with severe aortic regurgitation. N Engl J Med 2005;353:1342–9.

ELSEVIER
SAUNDERS

Heart Failure Clin 2 (2006) 473–482

HEART
FAILURE
CLINICS

Regurgitant Lesions of the Aortic and Mitral Valves: Considerations in Determining the Ideal Timing of Surgical Intervention

Edmund A. Bermudez, MD, MPH[a,b], William H. Gaasch, MD[a,c],*

[a]Lahey Clinic, Burlington, MA, USA
[b]Tufts University School of Medicine, Boston, MA, USA
[c]University of Massachusetts Medical School, Worcester, MA, USA

The optimal timing of corrective surgery for chronic severe aortic or mitral regurgitation depends on an appreciation of (1) the natural history of the lesion, particularly the changes of left ventricular (LV) size and function and the development of cardiac symptoms; and (2) the risks accompanying surgery, particularly the perioperative morbidity and mortality and the potential long-term complications of prosthetic heart valve implantation [1].

The left ventricle responds to the volume load of aortic or mitral regurgitation with a series of compensatory adaptations, primarily an increase in end-diastolic volume. As ventricular enlargement and hypertrophy develop, there is an increase in chamber compliance that accommodates the increased volume without a concomitant increase in LV end-diastolic pressure. The large diastolic volume provides a mechanism for the left ventricle to eject a large total stroke volume and thereby maintain a normal forward stroke volume despite a significant regurgitant volume. This is accomplished through myocardial fiber rearrangement and the addition of new sarcomeres. As a result, preload at the level of the myocyte (ie, sarcomere length) remains normal or near normal and contractile function is preserved. Thus, the enhanced total stroke volume is achieved through normal performance of each contractile unit around an enlarged circumference. Because of these adaptive changes, LV ejection performance remains normal.

Despite these similarities in structural change and function, there are significant differences between regurgitant lesions of the aortic and mitral valves that deserve comment. In aortic regurgitation, the systolic pressure and wall stress (afterload) tends to be increased and there is a combination of volume overload and pressure overload. This contributes to a combination of eccentric and concentric LV hypertrophy. By contrast, in mitral regurgitation, systolic wall stress is normal and the pattern of hypertrophic is eccentric. As these hemodynamic lesions progress and surgical correction becomes a consideration, it appears that chronic mitral regurgitation is less forgiving than chronic aortic regurgitation and that different criteria for corrective surgery are required for the two lesions. Echocardiography is the primary technique for the evaluation and follow-up of LV size and function [2], but invasive hemodynamic assessment may be required in some patients.

The development of overt heart failure generally should prompt consideration of surgical intervention; however, more subtle symptoms such as mild or even moderate dyspnea or fatigue can be problematic. Such symptoms may be early signs of LV decompensation, or they may be related to physical deconditioning or other comorbidities. This distinction is important because a failure to diagnose cardiac symptoms may allow progression of the hemodynamic burden and eventually a suboptimal outcome. On the other

* Corresponding author. Department of Cardiovascular Medicine, Lahey Clinic, 41 Mall Road, Burlington, MA 01805.

E-mail address: william.h.gaasch@lahey.org (W.H. Gaasch).

1551-7136/06/$ - see front matter © 2007 Elsevier Inc. All rights reserved.
doi:10.1016/j.hfc.2006.09.008

heartfailure.theclinics.com

hand, a failure to recognize noncardiac causes of dyspnea or fatigue may lead to unnecessary surgery. An objective assessment of exercise tolerance or measurement of plasma natriuretic peptide may provide useful information in some patients, but if limiting symptoms are not present, then it may be prudent to adapt a posture of watchful waiting with periodic re-evaluation. If surgery is indicated, then consideration must be given to potential surgical risks and the long-term problems associated with prosthetic heart valves and to the wishes and expectations of the patient.

Corrective surgery is indicated when severe aortic or mitral regurgitation is responsible for disabling symptoms or there is evidence that an increasing hemodynamic burden is affecting LV systolic function.

Aortic regurgitation

The severity of aortic insufficiency is readily assessed by echocardiography. An integrative approach is usually applied using all information from the echocardiographic study to arrive at a coherent assessment severity and should routinely include a careful two-dimensional assessment of the aortic valve, aorta, and LV chamber size and function.

Parameters for the grading of aortic regurgitation by echocardiography have been published (Table 1) [3]. Color flow imaging of the regurgitant jet provides important clues to the severity. The jet width and area in the parasternal views are important semiqualitative indicators of regurgitant severity. The size of the vena contracta provides a useful measure of severity when it exceeds 6 mm [4]. With these measures, the larger width or area, the greater the severity of regurgitation. Supportive signs of severe aortic regurgitation include a short pressure half-time of the aortic regurgitant signal, holodiastolic flow reversal in the descending thoracic aorta, and at least moderate LV enlargement [3]. A volumetric assessment [5] can be made by comparing aortic stroke volume to that of another uninvolved valve.

Hemodynamic assessment at cardiac catheterization can be used when noninvasive techniques fail to provide confident results [6]. Quantitative left ventriculography can be used to calculate regurgitant volumes and regurgitant fraction. Total stroke volume can be obtained by a careful angiographic assessment of end-diastolic and end-systolic volumes. When forward stroke volume (obtained from thermodilution or Fick cardiac output techniques) is subtracted from total stroke volume, regurgitant volume is derived. Further division by the total stroke volume results in the regurgitant fraction. A regurgitant fraction exceeding 50% is consistent with severe aortic insufficiency. Coronary angiography is performed to assess the status of the coronary arteries in patients at risk before surgical intervention.

Timing of surgical intervention

The prognosis of patients who have significant aortic insufficiency has been shown to be related to the presence of heart failure symptoms. In a study encompassing 246 patients followed conservatively with severe or moderately severe insufficiency, those who had New York Heart Association (NYHA) class III or IV heart failure had an annual mortality of 25%, whereas those who had class II heart failure had an annual mortality of 6% [7]. Surgery significantly reduced overall cardiovascular mortality. The presence of significant symptoms of heart failure or angina in other studies indicates high annual mortality rates ($>10\%$) in those treated conservatively [8,9].

Aortic valve surgery is indicated in patients who have normal LV function when NYHA class III or IV heart failure symptoms are present [10]. When milder symptoms are present, however, it is often unclear whether symptoms are cardiac in origin. Exercise stress testing may provide helpful information in such patients [11]. When marked LV enlargement (exceeding 75 mm at end-diastole) is present or when ejection fraction (EF) is borderline (50%–55%), however, the presence of even mild symptoms should prompt a consideration of surgical correction.

The aforementioned applies chiefly to patients who have chronic aortic insufficiency. Patients who have acute severe insufficiency invariably present with advanced symptomatology (pulmonary edema or cardiogenic shock) and often have normal LV systolic function, tachycardia, and normal LV chamber sizes. In these settings, compensatory mechanisms are often inadequate and poor outcomes are seen without prompt surgical intervention. Therefore, nearly all patients who have symptomatic severe aortic insufficiency, whether chronic or acute, should be considered candidates for surgical correction [12].

Surgical correction of symptomatic severe aortic insufficiency usually produces improvement in symptoms irrespective of the state of the left ventricle. In a small study of symptomatic patients

Table 1
Echocardiographic grading of aortic regurgitation

	Mild	Moderate	Severe
Specific signs for AR severity	Central jet width <25% of LVOT	Signs of AR greater than mild present but no criteria for severe AR	Central jet width ≥65% of LVOT
	Vena contracta <0.3 cm[a] No or brief early diastolic flow reversal in descending aorta		Vena contracta >0.6 cm[a]
Supportive signs (milliseconds)	Pressure half-time >500	Intermediate values	Pressure half-time <200
	Normal LV size[b]		Holodiastolic aortic flow reversal in descending aorta Moderate or greater LV enlargement[c]

Quantitative parameters[d]		Mild to moderate	Moderate to severe	
R Vol (mL/beat)[e]	<30	30–44	45–59	≥60
RF (%)	<30	30–39	40–49	≥50
EROA (cm2)[e]	<0.10	0.10–0.19	0.20–0.29	≥0.30

Abbreviations: AR, aortic regurgitation; EROA, effective regurgitant orifice area; LVOT, LV outflow tract; R Vol, regurgitant volume; RF, regurgitant fraction.

[a] At a Nyquist limit of 50–60 cm/s.

[b] LV size applied only to chronic lesions. Normal two-dimensional measurements: LV minor-axis <2.8 cm/m^2.

[c] In the absence of other etiologies of LV dilatation.

[d] Quantitative parameters can help subcalssify the moderate regurgitation group into mild-to-moderate and moderate-to-severe regurgitation as shown. Caution should be utilized when interpreting non-normalized volumes in isolation.

[e] Consider body size (body surface area).

Data from Zoghbi WA, Enriquez-Sarano M, Foster E, et al. Recommendations for evaluation of the severity of native valvular regurgitation with two-dimensional and Doppler echocardiography. J Am Soc Echocardiogr 2003;16: 777–802.

who had a mean preoperative EF of 45%, most had a decrease in symptoms and a postoperative increase in LV function (mean postoperative EF, 59%) [13]. Likewise, symptomatic patients who have mild or moderate LV dysfunction also benefit from corrective aortic valve surgery. Patients who have severe LV dysfunction or class IV symptoms have increased mortality rates and less chance of complete functional recovery postoperatively [14]. These patients often present difficult management issues because irreversible ventricular dysfunction may be present. Although perioperative risk is high in such patients, aortic valve surgery often provides a better alternative than medical therapy alone. In a study from the Mayo Clinic involving 450 patients who underwent aortic valve surgery for chronic aortic insufficiency, approximately 10% had LV EF levels below 35%. In such patients,

operative mortality was 14%; however, the LV EF increased by 4.9 percentage units after surgery, and most patients had prolonged survival without progression to heart failure. Thus, even though a controlled trial has not been performed, it can be recommended that such patients should not be denied the potential benefits of surgery [15]. A period of intense medical treatment to relieve the signs and symptoms of heart failure is warranted before surgical correction.

Asymptomatic patients

Some controversy exists regarding surgery for severe aortic regurgitation among asymptomatic individuals, particularly when LV systolic function is normal. LV size by echocardiography at end-diastole and end-systole has been recommended as a guide for recommending surgical intervention. Severe LV dilatation (LV end-diastolic dimension >75 mm) or systolic dysfunction (LV end-systolic dimension >55 mm) appears to represent high-risk patients who have an increased incidence of adverse outcomes without intervention [1,16]. Despite the lack of large-scale studies evaluating patients who have asymptomatic severe aortic insufficiency, conventional wisdom indicates that LV EF and end-systolic dimension are important predictors of survival and LV function following surgical correction [16]. Thus, an EF less than 50% or an end-systolic dimension greater than 55 mm can be considered an indication for aortic valve replacement in an asymptomatic patient. Patients who have moderately severe dilatation (LV end-diastolic dimension >70–75 mm), however, have been shown to have acceptable outcomes with conservative management [17], suggesting that end-diastolic size alone is not a strong indication for aortic valve replacement.

Serial monitoring is required in patients who have severe aortic insufficiency but who remain asymptomatic and do not yet meet criteria for surgical correction [18]. Patients who have a declining EF represent a subgroup at higher risk, and careful monitoring is mandatory [19]. In addition, some patients who develop systolic dysfunction do so without premonitory symptom development [20]. Therefore, in addition to serial follow-up for symptom evaluation, objective evidence by echocardiography is invaluable to identify asymptomatic patients who have LV dysfunction in whom surgical intervention is appropriate.

Management

An algorithm to guide timing of surgery in chronic severe aortic insufficiency has been developed (Fig. 1) [1]. In essence, all patients who have symptoms (functional class III or IV) or have LV dysfunction irrespective of symptoms should undergo corrective aortic valve surgery. Serial noninvasive monitoring is mandatory for the asymptomatic patients who do not have resting ventricular dysfunction or are not yet candidates for correction.

Mitral regurgitation

In a similar fashion as aortic insufficiency, an integrative approach is recommended when using echocardiography to assess the severity of mitral regurgitation [3]. The combination of two-dimensional color and spectral Doppler measurements and quantitative parameters aides in identifying severe mitral regurgitation in a more accurate and reproducible fashion. An application of specific and supportive parameters in mitral regurgitation is shown in Table 2. It should be recognized that chronic severe mitral insufficiency rarely exists without LV enlargement, so the presence of chronic severe mitral insufficiency should be questioned if the left ventricle is not enlarged. Likewise, the diagnosis of chronic severe mitral insufficiency should be questioned if left atrial enlargement is not present.

Color flow Doppler parameters can help to identify severe mitral insufficiency. Because the regurgitant jet area lacks accuracy, especially when the jet is eccentric, it should not be used as a single measure of severity [21]. Significant mitral regurgitation is likely present, however, when large jets penetrate the pulmonary veins and systolic flow reversal is seen. Measurement of the vena contracta may provide a more specific sign of severity, especially when measurements exceed 0.6 to 0.8 cm in long-axis views [22,23]. Care should be taken to avoid making this measurement in the apical two-chamber view because the vena contracta may be erroneously wide along the coaptation margins. Although measurement of the vena contracta works well with central or eccentric jets, multiple jets create fundamental problems with this technique.

Spectral Doppler measurements provide important adjunctive information to indicate severe mitral regurgitation. Pulmonary vein systolic flow reversal is a specific sign of hemodynamically severe regurgitation when seen in more than one pulmonary vein [24]. This finding is more reliable in acute or subacute than in chronic mitral insufficiency (it depends on left atrial compliance, and so forth). The height of the mitral E velocity is greater than the A wave velocity in severe mitral regurgitation and is usually greater than 1.2 cm/s. An A wave–dominant pattern virtually excludes severe mitral insufficiency [25]. Other supportive information of severe insufficiency is a dense, triangular, early peaking mitral-insufficient envelope on continuous wave Doppler sampling.

Quantitative methods can be used to assess the severity of mitral insufficiency. Calculation of stroke volumes in a similar manner as described previously for aortic regurgitation enable one to calculate regurgitant volume, regurgitant fraction, and regurgitant orifice area. Studies confirm the validity of this method to assess the severity of

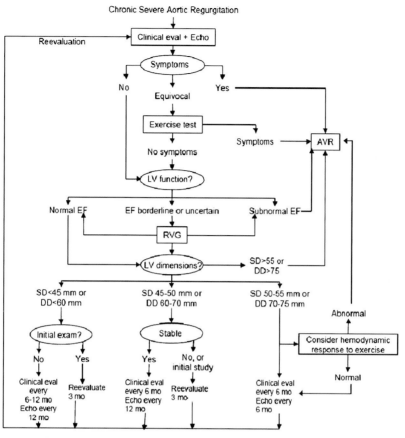

Fig. 1. Timing of surgery for aortic regurgitation. AVR, aortic valve replacement; Echo, echocardiography; DD, end-diastolic dimension; RVG, radionuclide ventriculography; SD, end-systolic dimension. (*Adapted from* Bonow RO, Carabello B, de Leon AC Jr, et al. ACC/AHA guidelines for the management of patients with valvular heart disease: a report of the American College of Cardiology/American Heart Association Task Force on Practice Guidelines (Committee on Management of Patients with Valvular Heart Disease). J Am Coll Cardiol 1998;32:1510; with permission.)

mitral insufficiency [26]. The proximal isovelocity surface area method has been validated and appears to be most accurate with central jets arising from circular orifices [26]. Regurgitant flow and an effective regurgitant orifice area (EROA) can be derived. An EROA of 0.4 cm^2 or greater is consistent with severe mitral insufficiency.

Hemodynamic evaluation at cardiac catheterization is used when clinical and noninvasive measures are disparate or inconclusive. Semiquantitative and quantitative measures are used to assess for severe insufficiency [6]. In a manner similar to that described for aortic insufficiency, regurgitant volumes and fractions can be derived, with regurgitant fractions exceeding 50% signifying severe mitral insufficiency.

Timing of surgical intervention

Factors predicting adverse outcomes after surgery include LV end-systolic dimension, EF, and the presence of atrial fibrillation [27]. Other measures of severe mitral insufficiency (ie, EROA) were recently evaluated prospectively and may help refine the definition of an optimal time for surgery [28].

The etiology of severe mitral insufficiency appears to impact prognosis. Those having primary leaflet abnormalities appear to have a more favorable outcome with surgical intervention. By contrast, those who have secondary insufficiency tend to have a prognosis that primarily depends on the underlying process. For example, ischemic or functional mitral insufficiency is associated

Table 2
Echocardiographic grading of mitral regurgitation

	Mild	Moderate	Severe
Specific signs of severity	Small central jet $<4\ cm^2$ or $<20\%$ of LA area[a]	Signs of MR greater than mild present but no criteria for severe MR	Vena contracta width $>7\ cm$ with large central MR jet (area $>40\%$ of LA) or with a wall-impinging jet of any size, swirling in LA[a]
	Vena contracta width $<0.3\ cm$ No or minimal flow convergence[b]		Large flow convergence[b] Systolic reversal in pulmonary veins Prominent flail MV leaflet or ruptured papillary muscle
Supportive signs	Systolic dominant flow in pulmonary veins A-wave dominant mitral inflow[c] Soft density, parabolic CW Doppler MR signal Normal LV siz[e]	Intermediate signs/findings	Dense, triangular CW Doppler MR jet E-wave dominant mitral inflow (E $>1.2\ m/s$)[c] Enlarged LV and LA size[d] (particularly when normal LV function is present)

Quantitative parameters[f]		Mild to moderate	Moderate to severe	
R Vol (mL/beat)[g]	<30	30–44	45–59	≥ 60
RF (%)	<30	30–39	40–49	≥ 50
EROA (cm^2)[g]	<0.20	0.20–0.29	0.30–0.39	≥ 0.4

Abbreviations: CW, continuous wave; EROA, effective regurgitant orifice area; LA, left atrium; MR, mitral regurgitation; MV, mitral valve; R Vol, regurgitant volume; RF, regurgitant fraction.

[a] At a Nyquist limit of 50–60 cm/s.

[b] Minimal and large flow convergence defined as a flow convergence radius of $<0.4\ cm$ and $\leq 0.9\ cm$ for central jets, respectively, with a baseline shift at a Nyquist of 40 cm/s; cut-offs for eccentric jets are higher and should be angle corrected.

[c] Usually >50 years of age or in condition of impaired relaxation, in the absence of mitral stenosis or other causes of elevated LA pressure.

[d] In the absence of other etiologies of LV and LA dilatation and acute MR.

[e] LV size applied only to chronic lesions. Normal two-dimensional measurements: LV minor axis $\leq 2.8\ cm/m^2$, LV end-diastolic volume $\leq 82\ mL/m^2$, maximal LA anteroposterior diameter $\leq 2.8\ cm/m^2$, maximal LA volume $\leq 36\ mL/m^2$.

[f] Quantitative parameters can help subclassify the moderate regurgitation group into mild-to-moderate and moderate-to-severe as shown.

[g] Consider body size (body surface area).

Data from Zoghbi WA, Enriquez-Sarano M, Foster E, et al. Recommendations for evaluation of the severity of native valvular regurgitation with two-dimensional and Doppler echocardiography. J Am Soc Echocardiogr 2003;16: 777–802.

with higher operative mortality, decreased survival, and a higher incidence of heart failure post surgery [29]. Here, the discussion centers on chronic mitral insufficiency originating from organic leaflet dysfunction.

Modern surgical methods generally involve either mitral valve replacement with preservation of the subvalvular apparatus or mitral valve repair [30]. When mitral valve replacement is performed, removal of the chordal apparatus is no longer performed, if possible. When the subvalvular apparatus is preserved during surgical replacement, postoperative LV function and survival are significantly improved compared with the result obtained when the mitral apparatus is disrupted [31,32]. It appears that preservation of the mitral apparatus may assist in the maintenance of a favorable LV geometry to favorably impact postoperative ventricular function.

Mitral valve repair is favored over valve replacement in almost all cases when feasible, and its attendant potential problems are avoided. Therefore, the issue of anticoagulation and the potential for future prosthetic failure can be avoided. Furthermore, mitral repair preserves the entire mitral apparatus, which is associated with superior postoperative survival and LV function [30]. The reoperation rates for mitral valve replacement and repair appear to be similar, with a reoperation rate approaching 10% by 10 years for those undergoing repair [33,34].

The feasibility of repair versus replacement can be assessed echocardiographically with transthoracic or transesophageal methods [29]. Repair is usually feasible when limited calcification of the leaflets or annulus is present, limited prolapse of only one leaflet exists, or when pure annular dilatation or valvular perforation is present. Replacement may be required if extensive calcification, severe prolapse, infection, or subvalvular involvement is seen [35,36].

Symptomatic patients who have chronic severe mitral insufficiency should be considered candidates for surgical intervention [37]. Patients who have normal LV function and little or no chamber enlargement can be candidates for surgery even when only mild symptoms are present, particularly when mitral valve repair is feasible [38]. Mitral valve surgery is also recommended when mild to moderate LV dysfunction is present (EF, 30%–55%) or when end-systolic dimension exceeds 45 mm [39]. Suboptimal outcome is more likely when severe LV dysfunction is present (EF <30% or end-systolic dimension >55 mm) [40]. Surgery is still reasonable, particularly if repair is feasible, whether a primary leaflet abnormality or functional insufficiency is present [14].

Asymptomatic patients

Despite the absence of symptoms, patients who have chronic severe mitral regurgitation and echocardiographic indicators of LV dysfunction are candidates for mitral valve surgery [41]. Indicators of ventricular dysfunction include a reduction in EF to less than 55% to 60% and an end-systolic dimension exceeding 45 mm [16,41].

Although mitral valve repair is preferred, a survival advantage can be expected whether repair or replacement is performed [38,42].

Some lack of agreement exists regarding surgical intervention in those who do not have indicators of LV dysfunction (EF > 60% or end-systolic dimension <40 mm). When atrial fibrillation or pulmonary hypertension (pulmonary artery systolic pressure > 50 mm Hg at rest or > 60 mm Hg with exercise) is present, however, early surgery is considered, especially if repair is feasible [27,43]. This recommendation is supported by evidence suggesting that atrial fibrillation independently predicts cardiac death and that a concomitant surgical maze procedure may prevent future events with the restoration of normal sinus rhythm [44–46]. In the absence of these factors, asymptomatic patients who have normal LV function should be followed closely with noninvasive studies. More recently, prospective studies have suggested that asymptomatic patients who have an EROA exceeding 0.4 cm^2 have a more favorable outcome with mitral valve surgery despite the absence of indicators for LV dysfunction because increasing EROA has implications for decreased survival with medical management [28]. Although these data are interesting, a single measurement to base referral for surgery is not advocated.

Management

The decision for surgery is based largely on the presence or absence of symptoms and the size and function of the left ventricle. If surgery is performed, then valve repair is preferred over replacement; if replacement is performed, then chordal preservation is always preferred. Patients who have echocardiographic indicators of LV dysfunction are candidates for surgery irrespective of symptomatology. When severe LV dysfunction is present, mitral valve surgery is reasonable when repair is feasible but can be problematic when replacement is attempted. When atrial fibrillation or pulmonary hypertension are present in asymptomatic individuals, early surgery should be considered, especially when repair is likely; otherwise, close monitoring is usually advocated with noninvasive measures (Fig. 2).

Summary

The timing of surgical intervention in native mitral and aortic regurgitation depends on several

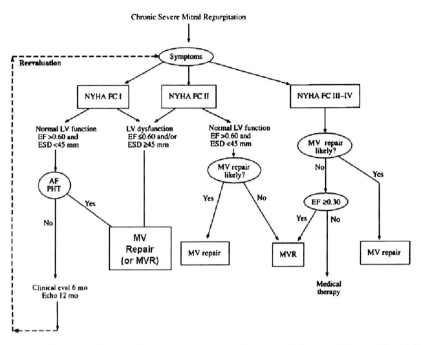

Fig. 2. Management strategy and timing of surgery in patients who have mitral regurgitation. AF, atrial fibriulation; Echo, echocardiography; ESD, end-systolic dimension; FC, functional class; MV, mitral valve; MVR, mitral valve replacement; PHT, pressure half-time. (*From* Bonow RO, Carabello B, de Leon AC Jr, et al. ACC/AHA guidelines for the management of patients with valvular heart disease: a report of the American College of Cardiology/American Heart Association Task Force on Practice Guidelines (Committee on Management of Patients with Valvular Heart Disease). J Am Coll Cardiol 1998;32:1533; with permission.)

factors including the severity of disease, the presence of symptoms, and the status of the left ventricle. In general, when significant symptoms attributable to the valvular lesion are present, outcome is more favorable when mechanical intervention is entertained. Regurgitant lesions, however, may remain relatively silent compared with stenotic lesions, and close attention should be paid to parameters indicative of impending ventricular failure, irrespective of the presence of symptoms. Therefore, noninvasive monitoring is invaluable for determining the most optimal time for surgical referral of these patients. Best clinical judgment and patient preference, however, remain important variables in the equation to determine individual therapeutic strategies.

References

[1] Bonow RO, Carabello B, de Leon AC, et al. ACC/ AHA guidelines for the management of patients with valvular heart disease. Executive summary. A report of the American College of Cardiology/ American Heart Association Task Force on

Practice Guidelines (Committee on Management of Patients with Valvular Heart Disease). J Am Coll Cardiol 1998;32:1486–588.

[2] Cheitlin MD, Armstrong WF, Aurigemma GP, et al. ACC/AHA/ASE 2003 guideline update for the clinical application of echocardiography—summary article: a report of the American College of Cardiology/American Heart Association Task Force on Practice Guidelines (ACC/AHA/ASE Committee to Update the 1997 Guidelines for the Clinical Application of Echocardiography). J Am Coll Cardiol 2003;42:954–70.

[3] Zoghbi WA, Enriquez-Sarano M, Foster E, et al. Recommendations for evaluation of the severity of native valvular regurgitation with two-dimensional and Doppler echocardiography. J Am Soc Echocardiogr 2003;16:777–802.

[4] Tribouilloy CM, Enriquez-Sarano M, Bailey KR, et al. Assessment of severity of aortic regurgitation using the width of the vena contracta: a clinical color Doppler imaging study. Circulation 2000;102: 558–64.

[5] Enriquez-Sarano M, Seward JB, Bailey KR, et al. Effective regurgitant orifice area: a noninvasive Doppler development of an old hemodynamic concept. J Am Coll Cardiol 1994;23:443–51.

[6] Kern MJ. The cardiac catheterization handbook. 4th edition. St. Louis (MO): Mosby Year Book; 2003.

[7] Dujardin KS, Enriquez-Sarano M, Schaff HV, et al. Mortality and morbidity of aortic regurgitation in clinical practice. A long-term follow-up study. Circulation 1999;99:1851–7.

[8] Aronow WS, Ahn C, Kronzon I, et al. Prognosis of patients with heart failure and unoperated severe aortic valvular regurgitation and relation to ejection fraction. Am J Cardiol 1994;74:286–8.

[9] Ishii K, Hirota Y, Suwa M, et al. Natural history and left ventricular response in chronic aortic regurgitation. Am J Cardiol 1996;78:357–61.

[10] Klodas E, Enriquez-Sarano M, Tajik AJ, et al. Optimizing timing of surgical correction in patients with severe aortic regurgitation: role of symptoms. J Am Coll Cardiol 1997;30:746–52.

[11] Wahi S, Haluska B, Pasquet A, et al. Exercise echocardiography predicts development of left ventricular dysfunction in medically and surgically treated patients with asymptomatic severe aortic regurgitation. Heart 2000;84:606–14.

[12] Nkomo VT. Indications for surgery for aortic regurgitation. Curr Cardiol Rep 2003;5:105–9.

[13] Carabello BA, Usher BW, Hendrix GH, et al. Predictors of outcome for aortic valve replacement in patients with aortic regurgitation and left ventricular dysfunction: a change in the measuring stick. J Am Coll Cardiol 1987;10:991–7.

[14] Carabello BA. Is it ever too late to operate on the patient with valvular heart disease? J Am Coll Cardiol 2004;44:376–83.

[15] Chaliki HP, Mohty D, Avierinos JF, et al. Outcomes after aortic valve replacement in patients with severe aortic regurgitation and markedly reduced left ventricular function. Circulation 2002;106:2687–93.

[16] Carabello BA, Crawford FA Jr. Valvular heart disease. N Engl J Med 1997;337:32–41.

[17] Tarasoutchi F, Grinberg M, Spina GS, et al. Ten-year clinical laboratory follow-up after application of a symptom-based therapeutic strategy to patients with severe chronic aortic regurgitation of predominant rheumatic etiology. J Am Coll Cardiol 2003;41:1316–24.

[18] Borer JS, Bonow RO. Contemporary approach to aortic and mitral regurgitation. Circulation 2003;108:2432–8.

[19] Bonow RO, Lakatos E, Maron BJ, et al. Serial long-term assessment of the natural history of asymptomatic patients with chronic aortic regurgitation and normal left ventricular systolic function. Circulation 1991;84:1625–35.

[20] Scognamiglio R, Rahimtoola SH, Fasoli G, et al. Nifedipine in asymptomatic patients with severe aortic regurgitation and normal left ventricular function. N Engl J Med 1994;331:689–94.

[21] Enriquez-Sarano M, Tajik AJ, Bailey KR, et al. Color flow imaging compared with quantitative Doppler assessment of severity of mitral regurgitation: influence of eccentricity of jet and mechanism of regurgitation. J Am Coll Cardiol 1993;21:1211–9.

[22] Hall SA, Brickner ME, Willett DL, et al. Assessment of mitral regurgitation severity by Doppler color flow mapping of the vena contracta. Circulation 1997;95:636–42.

[23] Heinle SK, Hall SA, Brickner ME, et al. Comparison of vena contracta width by multiplane transesophageal echocardiography with quantitative Doppler assessment of mitral regurgitation. Am J Cardiol 1998;81:175–9.

[24] Pu M, Griffin BP, Vandervoort PM, et al. The value of assessing pulmonary venous flow velocity for predicting severity of mitral regurgitation: a quantitative assessment integrating left ventricular function. J Am Soc Echocardiogr 1999;12:736–43.

[25] Thomas L, Foster E, Schiller NB. Peak mitral inflow velocity predicts mitral regurgitation severity. J Am Coll Cardiol 1998;31:174–9.

[26] Pu M, Prior DL, Fan X, et al. Calculation of mitral regurgitant orifice area with use of a simplified proximal convergence method: initial clinical application. J Am Soc Echocardiogr 2001;14:180–5.

[27] Lung B, Gohlke-Barwolf C, Tornos P, et al. Recommendations on the management of the asymptomatic patient with valvular heart disease. Eur Heart J 2002;23:1252–66.

[28] Enriquez-Sarano M, Avierinos JF, Messika-Zeitoun D, et al. Quantitative determinants of the outcome of asymptomatic mitral regurgitation. N Engl J Med 2005;352:875–83.

[29] Enriquez-Sarano M, Freeman WK, Tribouilloy CM, et al. Functional anatomy of mitral regurgitation: accuracy and outcome implications of transesophageal echocardiography. J Am Coll Cardiol 1999;34:1129–36.

[30] Enriquez-Sarano M, Schaff HV, Orszulak TA, et al. Valve repair improves the outcome of surgery for mitral regurgitation. A multivariate analysis. Circulation 1995;91:1022–8.

[31] Tischler MD, Cooper KA, Rowen M, et al. Mitral valve replacement versus mitral valve repair. A Doppler and quantitative stress echocardiographic study. Circulation 1994;89:132–7.

[32] Horskotte D, Schulte HD, Bircks W, et al. The effect of chordal preservation on late outcome after mitral valve replacement: a randomized study. J Heart Valve Dis 1993;2:150–8.

[33] Gillinov AM, Cosgrove DM, Lytle BW, et al. Reoperation for failure of mitral valve repair. J Thorac Cardiovasc Surg 1997;113:467–73 [discussion: 473–5].

[34] Mohty D, Orszulak TA, Schaff HV, et al. Very long-term survival and durability of mitral valve repair for mitral valve prolapse. Circulation 2001;104:II-7.

[35] Hellemans IM, Pieper EG, Ravelli AC, et al. Prediction of surgical strategy in mitral valve regurgitation based on echocardiography. Interuniversity Cardiology Institute of the Netherlands. Am J Cardiol 1997;79:334–8.

[36] Chaudhry FA, Upadya SP, Singh VP, et al. Identifying patients with degenerative mitral regurgitation for mitral valve repair and replacement: a transesophageal echocardiographic study. J Am Soc Echocardiogr 2004;17:988–94.

[37] Otto CM. Timing of surgery in mitral regurgitation. Heart 2003;89:100–5.

[38] Enriquez-Sarano M, Tajik AJ, Schaff HV, et al. Echocardiographic prediction of survival after surgical correction of organic mitral regurgitation. Circulation 1994;90:830–7.

[39] Bonow RO, Nikas D, Elefteriades JA. Valve replacement for regurgitant lesions of the aortic or mitral valve in advanced left ventricular dysfunction. Cardiol Clin 1995;13:73–85.

[40] Otto CM. Clinical practice. Evaluation and management of chronic mitral regurgitation. N Engl J Med 2001;345:740–6.

[41] Gaasch WH, John RM, Aurigemma GP. Managing asymptomatic patients with chronic mitral regurgitation. Chest 1995;108:842–7.

[42] Enriquez-Sarano M, Tajik AJ, Schaff HV, et al. Echocardiographic prediction of left ventricular function after correction of mitral regurgitation: results and clinical implications. J Am Coll Cardiol 1994;24:1536–43.

[43] Grigioni F, Avierinos JF, Ling LH, et al. Atrial fibrillation complicating the course of degenerative mitral regurgitation: determinants and long-term outcome. J Am Coll Cardiol 2002;40:84–92.

[44] Schaff HV, Dearani JA, Daly RC, et al. Cox-Maze procedure for atrial fibrillation: Mayo Clinic experience. Semin Thorac Cardiovasc Surg 2000;12:30–7.

[45] Kobayashi J, Sasako Y, Bando K, et al. Eight-year experience of combined valve repair for mitral regurgitation and maze procedure. J Heart Valve Dis 2002;11:165–71 [discussion: 171–2].

[46] Handa N, Schaff HV, Morris JJ, et al. Outcome of valve repair and the Cox maze procedure for mitral regurgitation and associated atrial fibrillation. J Thorac Cardiovasc Surg 1999;118:628–35.

ELSEVIER
SAUNDERS

Heart Failure Clin 2 (2006) 483–487

Index

Note: Page numbers of article titles are in **boldface** type.

Moving?

Make sure your subscription moves with you!

To notify us of your new address, find your **Clinics Account Number** (located on your mailing label above your name), and contact customer service at:

E-mail: elspcs@elsevier.com

800-654-2452 (subscribers in the U.S. & Canada)
407-345-4000 (subscribers outside of the U.S. & Canada)

Fax number: 407-363-9661

Elsevier Periodicals Customer Service
6277 Sea Harbor Drive
Orlando, FL 32887-4800

*To ensure uninterrupted delivery of your subscription, please notify us at least 4 weeks in advance of move.